D0418532

Helen McGuinness

INDIAN HEAD
MASSAGE

second edition

Hodder Arnold

A MEMBER OF THE HODDER HEADLINE GROUP

Orders: please contact Bookpoint Ltd, 130 Milton Park, Abingdon, Oxon OX14 4SB. Telephone: (44) 01235 827720. Fax: (44) 01235 400454. Lines are open from 9.00 – 5.00, Monday to Saturday, with a 24 hour message answering service. You can also order through our website www.hoddereducation.co.uk

British Library Cataloguing in Publication Data
A catalogue record for this title is available from the British Library

ISBN-10: 0 340 81473 X
ISBN-13: 978 0 340 81473 4

First Edition published 2000
Second Edition published 2004
Impression number   10 9 8 7 6 5 4
Year   2007 2006

Copyright © 2000, 2004 Helen McGuinness

All rights reserved. No part of this publication may be reproduced or transmitted in any form or by any means, electronic or mechanical, including photocopy, recording, or any information storage and retrieval system, without permission in writing from the publisher or under licence from the Copyright Licensing Agency Limited. Further details of such licences (for reprographic reproduction) may be obtained from the Copyright Licensing Agency Limited, 90 Tottenham Court Road, London W1T 4LP.

Cover photo from James Newell Photographer
Typeset by Fakenham Photosetting Limited, Fakenham, Norfolk
Printed in Dubai for Hodder Arnold, an imprint of Hodder Education, a member of the Hodder Headline Group, 338 Euston Road, London NW1 3BH

Contents

Acknowledgements

I would like to acknowledge and thank the following people for their support in the writing of this book:

My husband Mark for his considerable help and contributions, for his constant love and support, and especially for inspiring and encouraging me to write this book; my parents Roy and Val for their positive encouragement and constant belief in my abilities; my dear friend Dee Chase for her valuable contributions and for her support and encouragement throughout the writing of this book; Dr Nathan Moss for his invaluable advice for Chapter 3 – Conditions Affecting the Head, Neck and Shoulders; Lisa Callaway for modelling for the photographs in Chapter 6; James Newell for taking the photographs; and finally all the Indian Head Massage students at the Holistic Training Centre who have encouraged me to write this book.

The publishers would like to thank the following individuals and institutions for permission to reproduce copyright material:

Nim Mengat – 7; Science Photo Library – 24, 25 (Folliculitis, Impetigo), 26, 27 (Tinea Capitis), 28, 29, 30; © The Cover Story/Corbis – 2; Wellcome Photo Library – 25 (Sycosis barbae), 27 (Tinea barbae).

Every effort has been made to obtain necessary permission with reference to copyright material. The publishers apologise if inadvertently any sources remain unacknowledged and will be glad to make the necessary arrangements at the earliest opportunity.

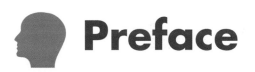

Preface

Originally developed as a family tradition in its country of origin, Indian Head Massage has grown in popularity from being a technique which was mainly practised on the head by families in India, to become a comprehensive holistic therapy skill that addresses the widespread problems of stress in the Western world.

This book is designed for those undertaking a professional qualification in Indian Head Massage and addresses all the generic skills and knowledge required for commercial practice and competence in the workplace.

Indian Head Massage has grown in popularity in the late part of the 1990s to become an integral part of Holistic Therapy course programmes in further education colleges and private training establishments.

This book is presented in a workbook format in order to help students to generate sufficient evidence to reach a competent level for commercial practice. It is also formulated to assist tutors in their course design and delivery and in assessment of candidates' essential knowledge required for competence.

Helen McGuinness

Introduction to Indian Head Massage

Massage has always been an important feature of Indian family life. Indian Head Massage is a treatment that has evolved from traditional techniques that have been practised in India as part of a family ritual for thousands of years.

By the end of this chapter, you will be able to relate the following to your work as a holistic therapist:

chapter contents

- The basic principles of Ayurveda
- The history and development of Indian Head Massage as a holistic therapy
- The benefits and effects of Indian Head Massage.

The History and Development of Indian Head Massage

The traditional art of Indian Head Massage is based on the ancient system of medicine known as Ayurveda, which has been practised in India for thousands of years.

Ayurveda

Ayurveda is recorded as the world's oldest Indian healing system. The word 'Ayurveda' comes from Sanskrit and means 'the science of life and longevity'. The Ayurvedic approach to health is the balance of body, mind and spirit, and the promotion of long life.

Ayurveda recommends the use of massage together with diet, herbs, cleansing, yoga, meditation and exercise.

The ancient texts say that the human life span should be around 100 years, and that all those years should be lived in total health, physically and emotionally. The whole aim of Ayurveda is in prevention, and with promoting positive health, beauty and long life.

The early Ayurvedic texts, dating back nearly 4,000 years, feature massage and the principles of holistic treatment, in that health results from harmony within one's self. The Ayur-Veda, a sacred book among

Hindus, written around 1800 BC, included massage amongst its Ayurvedic principles. The Hindus used techniques preserved in the Sanskrit texts 2,500 years ago, which detail the underlying principles of Ayurveda in maintaining balance in the body.

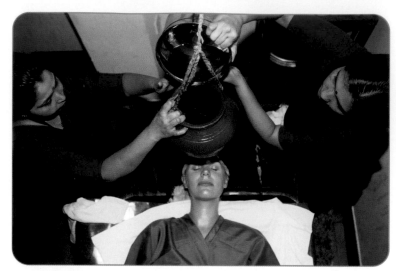

An Ayurvedic treatment

Ayurvedic principles

The Ayurvedic view of health is in physical, emotional and spiritual wellbeing and that health is maintained by the balance of three subtle life-giving forces or **doshas**: **Vata**, **Pitta** and **Kapha**. Each of the three doshas has a role to play in the body:

* **Vata** is the driving force, and relates mainly to the nervous system and the body's energy centre
* **Pitta** is fire and relates to metabolism, digestion, enzymes, acid and bile
* **Kapha** is related to water in the mucous membranes, phlegm, moisture, fat and lymphatics.

In Ayurveda, a person is seen as a unique individual made up of five primary elements: ether (space), air, fire, water and earth. When any of these elements are imbalanced in the environment, they will have an influence on how an individual feels. The foods we eat and the weather are just two of the influences on these elements.

While each individual is a composite of the five primary elements, certain elements are seen to have an ability to create various physiological functions.

* The elements combine with ether and air in dominance to form what is known in Ayurveda as **Vata**, which governs the principle of movement and therefore can be seen as the force which directs nerve impulses, circulation, respiration and elimination.
* The elements with fire and water in dominance combine to form **Pitta**, which is responsible for the process of transformation or metabolism. The transformation of foods into nutrition is an example of Pitta function.
* It is predominantly the elements of water and earth that combine to form **Kapha**, which is responsible for growth. It also offers protection, for example in the form of cerebro–spinal fluid, which protects the brain and the spinal column. The mucosal lining of the stomach is another example of the Kapha dosha protecting the tissues.

Characteristics of the three doshas

Each dosha possesses individual qualities and their increase or decrease in the system depends upon the antagonistic qualities of everything ingested.

- **Vata** is dry, cold, light, mobile, clear, rough and subtle.
- **Pitta** is slightly oily, hot, intense, light, fluid, free-flowing.
- **Kapha** is oily, cold, heavy, stable, smooth and soft.

- Both **Vata** and **Pitta** are light, and only **Kapha** is heavy.
- Both **Vata** and **Kapha** are cold, and only **Pitta** is hot.
- Both **Pitta** and **Kapha** are moist and oily, and only **Vata** is dry.

- Anything dry almost always increases Vata, anything hot increases Pitta and anything heavy increases Kapha.

The sub-doshas

Each of the three doshas has a sub-division of five aspects, each one controlling a function or system of the body. These are useful to know, as they can indicate which dosha is unbalanced.

Vata

- In general, Vata controls all movement in the body and mind, and is related directly to the nervous system
- Vata creates dryness in the body when too high and sluggishness when too low
- Together with Pitta, Vata controls the hormonal function. The other two doshas are inert without Vata.

The five sub-divisions that control various aspects of Vata are:

1 **Prana vayu** – controls inhalation, the other four vayus, the five senses, thinking, health and proper growth.
   Indications of imbalance: loss of senses, anxiety and worry, insomnia, dryness, emaciation, disease in general.

2 **Apana vayu** – controls elimination, sexual function, menstruation, downwards movements in the body, and disease.
   Indications of imbalance: constipation, menstrual problems, dryness, urinary problems: generally, all diseases are involved.

3 **Samana vayu** – controls movement of the digestive system and the solar plexus, and balances the prana and apana vayus.
   Indications of imbalance: upset digestion, indigestion, diarrhoea, malabsorption of nutrients, dryness.

4 **Udan vayu** – controls exhalation, speech and the upward movements in the body, growth as a child.

Indications of imbalance: problems with speech and the throat, weakness of will, general fatigue, lack of enthusiasm.

5   **Vyana vayu** – pervades the whole body as the nervous system, yet it controls heart function and circulation of blood.
Indications of imbalance: arthritis, nervousness, poor circulation, poor motor reflexes, problems with the joints, bone disorders, nervous disorders.

Pitta

- In general, Pitta is responsible for all metabolic processes. Pitta enables us to digest thoughts, feelings or food. Pitta controls all the heat disorders and relates to the fiery organs in the body and the blood. Together with Vata, it controls the hormonal function.
- Low Pitta will cause the whole metabolism to slow down and usually goes with high Kapha. Excess Pitta causes all kinds of heat-related disorders and inflammations.

The five sub-divisions that control various aspects of Pitta are:

1   **Alochaka pitta** – controls the ability to see and the digestion of what we see.
Indications of imbalance: eye problems and difficulties in digesting what we see.

2   **Sadaka pitta** – controls functions of the heart and the digestion of thoughts and emotions.
Indications of imbalance: heart failure, repressed emotions and feelings, excessive anger or unprocessed feelings.

3   **Pachaka pitta** – controls stomach digestion.
Indications of imbalance: ulcers, heartburn, cravings, indigestion.

4   **Ranjaka pitta** – controls liver/gall bladder digestion.
Indications of imbalance: anger, irritability, hostility, excessive bile, liver disorders, skin problems, toxic blood, anaemia.

5   **Bhrajaka pitta** – controls metabolism of the skin.
Indications of imbalance: all skin problems, acne, inflammation of the skin.

Kapha

- In general, Kapha is responsible for the stability of our body and mind. It is the principal cohesion of mind and body. Flexibility and growth are controlled by Kapha; moisture and fluid retention are maintained by it.
- When Kapha is too high it restricts Vata and subdues Pitta, thereby creating congestion on all levels.
- When Kapha is too low it results in dryness and ungrounded thoughts and actions.

1   **Tarpaka kapha** – controls fluids in the head, the sinuses and cerebral fluids.
Indications of imbalance: sinus problems, headaches, loss of smell.

2   **Bodhaka kapha** – controls taste and the cravings of taste, digestion and saliva.

Indications of imbalance: overeating and cravings for sweets, loss of taste, congestion in the throat and mouth areas.

3   **Avalambaka kapha** – controls lubrication and the fluids around the heart, lungs and upper back.
    Indications of imbalance: congestion in the lungs or heart, stiffness in the back and upper spine, lethargy.

4   **Kledaka kapha** – controls the lubrication of the digestive processes, maintains a balance with the Pitta's bile, provides mental lubrication.
    Indications of imbalance: bloated stomach, slow or congested digestion, excess mucus.

5   **Slesaka kapha** – controls the lubrication of the joints in the body, and aids in all movements.
    Indications of imbalance: swollen joints, stiff joints, painful movements.

The importance of Prana

- The secret of Ayurveda lies in *prana*, the vital force (pra = before, and ana = breath).
- In Ayurveda, strong prana is the source of good health.
- There are five major pranas in the human body to support all movement and bodily functions.
- The five pranas are normally called vayus. The descriptions of the pranas outlined below are not definitive, as they interrelate to each other and are very complex in their movements.

Prana vayu
This is the 'inward moving' air that is located in the head and the heart. It controls thinking, inhalation, emotions, sensory functioning, memory and receiving the cosmic prana from the sun (hot or solar prana). It provides the basic energy that moves us in life.

Apana vayu
This is the 'downward-moving' air seated in the colon. It controls all the processes of elimination including urine, sweat, menstruation, orgasm and defecation. The apana receives cosmic prana from the earth and moon (cool or lunar prana). It also rules the elimination of negative emotions and provides mental stability. It is the basis of our immune system and when disturbed is the cause of most diseases.

Udana vayu
This is the 'upward-moving' air located in the throat. It controls speech, connects us to the solar and lunar forces (sky and earth; masculine and feminine) and is responsible for spiritual development. Udana controls psychic powers and creative expression.

Samana vayu
This is known as the 'equalising or balancing' air. It is seated in the navel and controls the digestive system and harmonises the prana and apana. Samana also governs the digestion of air, emotions and feeling. It is hot and solar in nature.

Vyana vayu

This is called the 'pervading' or 'outward-moving' air. It is seated in the heart and yet pervades the whole body. It unites the other pranas and the tissues, and controls nerve and muscle action. It holds the body together and is responsible for all circulation in the body: food, blood and emotions. Vyana provides strength and stability to the body.

Balance and harmony of the three doshas

When the three doshas are well harmonised and balanced, good health and wellbeing will result. However, when there is imbalance or disharmony in the elements it can lead to various types of ailments.

The Ayurvedic concept of physical health revolves around the three doshas and the primary purpose is to maintain them in a balanced state, to prevent disease and disharmony. This theory is not unique to Indian medicine; the Yin and Yang theory in Chinese medicine and the Hippocrates theory in Greek medicine are also very similar.

Each individual is made up of unique proportions of Vata, Pitta and Kapha. The ratio of the doshas varies in each individual and, as Ayurveda sees each person as a special combination, that accounts for our diversity. Each individual's constitution is determined by the state of their parents' doshas at the time of conception; at birth, a person has the levels of the three doshas that are right for them. Life and all its forces and influences can cause the doshas to become unbalanced, which can lead to ill health.

Ayurveda offers a model to look at each individual as a unique make-up of the three doshas and it designs a treatment protocol to address a person's specific health challenges.

When any of the doshas becomes accumulated, Ayurveda will suggest specific lifestyle and nutritional guidelines to assist the individual in reducing the dosha that has become excessive. Also, herbal medicines will be suggested, to cure the imbalance and diseases.

Understanding the main principle of Ayurveda offers an explanation as to why one person responds differently to a treatment or diet than another and why individuals with the same disease may require different treatments and medication.

Massage in Indian family life

Traditionally, massage has always been an important feature of family life across the generations. In Indian traditions, the belief is that massage preserves the body's life force and energy, and is the most powerful way of relaxing and rejuvenating the body.

In India, it is customary for babies to be massaged every day from birth and to be massaged continually until they are three years old. This encourages the bonding process, keeps the babies healthy and happy and helps create a secure family environment.

From the age of six, children are taught to show love and respect by sharing a massage with family members.

It is considered compulsory for a bride and groom to receive a massage with chemicals and oils before marriage. This ceremonial massage is considered to help relax the bride and groom and to give them stamina and psychic strength, as well as to promote health and fertility. In India, it is also traditional to massage expectant mothers to help them cope with the physical and emotional demands of labour; massage is applied daily for a minimum of 40 days after the birth. Weekly massage is a family event in India and for the majority continues throughout life to old age.

The Indian Head Massage techniques practised today have evolved from traditional rituals of Indian family grooming. Over generations, Indian women have been taught by their mothers to massage coconut, sesame, olive, almond, herbal and mustard oils, buttermilk, and henna into their scalp, in order to maintain their hair in beautiful condition.

In India, barbers have developed a more stimulating and invigorating head massage, known as 'champi', to incorporate into their daily

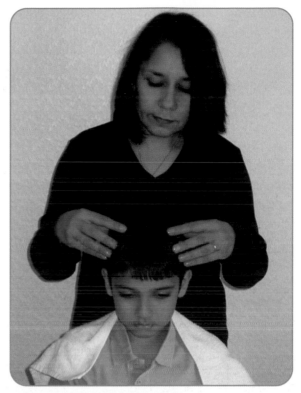

Indian Head Massage in family life

treatments, which leaves their clients feeling revitalised and alert. Their particular techniques are passed down through the generations, from barber father to barber son.

The original tradition of Indian Head Massage has therefore been passed on through the family generations, as Indian women have been taught the tradition of hair massage and grooming from their mothers and barbers' sons have learnt techniques from their fathers.

In India, head massage forms an integral part of family life and is often a ritual that is performed not only at home within families, but on street corners, on the beaches and in market places.

Indian Head Massage in the Western world

Despite being in existence on the Indian sub-continent for thousands of years, Indian Head Massage has only recently started to gain popularity in the West.

Indian Head Massage was originally designed for use on the head; today it is no longer confined only to the head area, and has been Westernised to include other parts of the body vulnerable to stress, such as the shoulders, upper arms and neck.

It is important to realise that there is an integral relationship between the head, neck, shoulders and upper arms and by incorporating these parts the treatment becomes more of a stress management treatment, rather than a treatment designed to stimulate the head and improve the hair growth and condition. Although the techniques are applied to the upper part of the body only (shoulders, upper arms, neck and head), collectively they represent a de-stressing programme for the whole body.

Indian Head Massage has therefore become a primary form of stress management treatment in the Western world.

Clients seeking relief from stress and tension often find Indian Head Massage a convenient form of treatment to receive in that:

- there is no need to undress
- it is quick and effective in terms of results
- it may be accessed anywhere, because of its portable nature.

Therapists find Indian Head Massage a convenient form of treatment to offer in that:

- no special resources are needed
- the techniques used are quick and effective
- clients with special needs (for example, a heavily pregnant client, or a client in a wheelchair) may receive treatment with the minimum fuss.

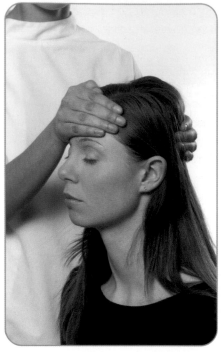

Indian Head Massage in the Western world

The Future of Indian Head Massage

Today, Indian Head Massage is one of the fastest-growing holistic therapies.

In 1996, in response to market demand for the skill, Indian Head Massage was first formalised into a Diploma qualification by VTCT (Vocational Training Charitable Trust). Other awarding bodies, such as ITEC (International Therapy Education Council), CIBTAC (Confederation of International Beauty Therapy and Cosmetology) and City and Guilds, have also developed qualifications in this field. Indian Head Massage is now being incorporated into the National Occupational Standards for both Hairdressing and Beauty Therapy at Level III. This is a significant development, in that what was previously a variable form of treatment passed down through Indian families has attracted a professional qualification with national and international standards in the health and beauty industry.

Indian Head Massage is now available in hairdressing and beauty salons, spas, health farms, health clinics, in the workplace/offices, at airports, on airlines, at conferences and exhibitions, on cruise liners and in private practice. Indian Head Massage owes its diversity of practice to both its versatility and accessibility.

Despite its diversity of development, there is still a significant potential for the practice of Indian Head

Massage to be widened in the market. Being a portable skill, *and* the perfect antidote to stress and tension, it is beneficial to all members of the community (from the young to the elderly).

A relatively untapped area of potential is in the corporate market. The treatment can be tailored to be offered within a lunch hour or break, and marketed as a stress management tool and preventive health care therapy.

Stress-related issues are responsible for around 60% of the 67 million working days lost each year, according to recent figures from the Health and Safety Executive. The development of Indian Head Massage in the workplace can help to reduce the harmful effects of stress, while energising and motivating the workforce.

The Effects and Benefits of Indian Head Massage

Although the techniques involved in Indian Head Massage involve only the upper part of the body, the potential benefits are widespread. It can be said that Indian Head Massage is a truly holistic therapy in that it has many physiological and psychological benefits; many clients comment on the fact that they feel as if their whole body is balanced after the treatment.

EFFECTS	BENEFITS
Increase in blood flow to the head, neck and shoulders	• Nourishes the tissues and encourages healing • Improves the circulation; the delivery of oxygen and nutrients is improved via the arterial circulation and the removal of wastes is hastened via the venous flow
Increased lymphatic flow to the head, neck and shoulders	• Aids the elimination of accumulated toxins and waste products • Reduces oedema • Stimulates immunity
Relaxes the muscle and nerve fibres of the head, neck and shoulders	• Relieves muscular tension and fatigue • Increases flexibility • Improves posture • Can help to relieve tension headaches and aches and pains
Reduces spasms, restrictions and adhesions in the muscle fibres	• Relieves pain and discomfort • Improves joint mobility
Decreases inflammation in the tissues	• Pain relief • Reduces stress placed on bones and joints
Decreases stimulation of the sympathetic nervous system	• Slows down and deepens breathing • Slows down the heart rate • Helps reduce blood pressure • Reduces stress and anxiety
Activates the parasympathetic nervous system	• Encourages the body to rest and relax • Helps promote sleep
Improves circulation to the skin and the hair	• Encourages cell regeneration

EFFECTS	BENEFITS
Increases circulation to the scalp	• Promotes healthy head growth • Helps improve the condition of the skin and hair
Relaxes and soothes tense eye muscles	• Helps relieve tired eyes and eyestrain • Brightens the eyes
Increases the supply of oxygen to the brain	• Helps relieve mental fatigue • Promotes clearer thinking • Improves concentration • Increases productivity
Stimulates the release of endorphins from the brain	• Helps relieve pain • Helps relieve emotional stress and repressed feelings • Elevates the mood – can help anxiety and depression
Encourages the release of stagnant energy and restores the energy flow to the body	• Creates a feeling of balance and calm

SELF-ASSESSMENT QUESTIONS

1 Indian Head Massage has evolved from

   a Sanskrit texts dating from 2,500 years ago

   b the sacred book of Ayur-Veda dating from 1800 BC

   c an Indian family tradition

   d the ancient system of Indian medicine, Ayurveda.

2 The Ayurvedic principle is that health is maintained by

   a having a regular Indian Head Massage

   b balancing of the three doshas

   c eating the correct diet

   d using special oils on the hair.

3 In Ayurveda, which of the following is a characteristic of the dosha Kapha?

   a dry

   b light

   c rough

   d heavy.

4 Which of the following statements is incorrect?

   a imbalances in the doshas can lead to ill health

   b each individual is made of the same proportions of Vata, Pitta and Kapha

   c life and all its forces and influences can cause the doshas to become unbalanced

   d each individual's constitution is determined by the state of their parents' doshas at the time of conception.

5 Which of the following statements is incorrect?

   a Indian Head Massage helps reduce stress and anxiety

   b Indian Head Massage decreases the release of endorphins from the brain

   c Indian Head Massage increases the blood flow to the head, neck and shoulders

   d Indian Head Massage helps relieve tired eyes and eyestrain.

2 Essential Anatomy and Physiology for Indian Head Massage

In order to understand the physiological effects of Indian Head Massage on the body, it is important for a holistic therapist to have a knowledge of essential anatomy and physiology to be able to carry out treatments safely and effectively. This chapter is devoted to the anatomy and physiology relevant to Indian Head Massage.

By the end of this chapter, you will be able to relate the following knowledge to your practice in Indian Head Massage:

chapter contents

- The structure and functions of the skin and hair
- Diseases and disorders in relation to skin and hair
- The bones of the head, neck and shoulders
- Muscles of the head, neck, upper back, shoulder and upper arms
- The blood flow relating to the head and neck
- The lymphatic drainage of the head and neck
- The nerve supply to the head and neck
- The mechanism of respiration.

The Skin

- The skin is the largest organ of the body and provides the therapeutic foundation for treatment.
- The skin provides more than just an external covering; it is a highly sensitive boundary between our bodies and the environment.
- A thorough knowledge of the structure and functions of the skin will help the therapist to treat clients more effectively.

Functions of the skin

The skin has several important functions:

Protection

- The skin acts like a physical barrier protecting the underlying tissues from abrasion. Keratin, a protein found in the skin, provides protection by waterproofing the skin's surface, helping to keep water in and out.
- The skin also provides limited protection from ultra-violet radiation through specialised cells called melanocytes found in the basal cell layer of the epidermis.
- The skin's acidic secretions (sweat and sebum), known as the **acid mantle**, act as a barrier against foreign agents such as bacteria and viruses.
- Fat cells in the subcutaneous layer of the skin help protect bones and major organs from injury.

Sensation

The skin is like an extension of the nervous system in that it receives stimuli such as pressure, pain and temperature from the external environment and brings this information to the central nervous system.

Heat regulation

The skin helps to regulate the body's temperature at a temperature of 37°C:

- when the body is losing too much heat, the blood capillaries near the skin's surface constrict to keep warmth in and closer to major organs
- when the body is too warm, the blood capillaries dilate to allow more blood to flow near the surface in order to cool the body
- the sweat glands also help to cool the body down through the production of sweat.

Excretion

The skin functions as a minor excretory system, eliminating waste through perspiration.

The eccrine glands of the skin produce sweat, which helps to remove from the skin waste materials such as urea, uric acid, ammonia and lactic acid.

Secretion

The specialised glands in the skin called the sebaceous glands secrete the oily substance sebum which flows onto the skin's surface, lubricating it and keeping it soft and pliable.

Storage

The skin acts as a storage depot for fat and water. About 15 per cent of the body's fluids are stored in the subcutaneous layer.

Absorption

The skin has limited absorption properties. Substances that can be absorbed by the epidermis are fat-soluble substances such as oxygen, carbon dioxide, fat-soluble vitamins and steroids, along with small amounts of water.

Vitamin D production

Located in the skin are molecules that are converted by the ultra-violet rays in sunlight to vitamin D. The vitamin D produced is then absorbed into the blood vessels and used by the body for the maintenance of bones and the absorption of calcium and phosphorus in the diet.

Structure of the skin

- Each client's skin varies in its colour, texture and condition.
- A client's skin can reflect their physiological as well as psychological state, and it is through touch that therapists can help to evaluate this information.
- Physiological signs of the skin may be shown by the client's colour and circulation, whereas psychological status may be reflected by muscular tightness.

There are two main layers of the skin:

- the **epidermis**, which is the outer thinner layer
- the **dermis**, which is the inner thicker layer.

Below the dermis is the **subcutaneous layer** which attaches to organs and tissues.

The epidermis

The epidermis is the most superficial layer of the skin and consists of five layers of cells:

- the horny layer (*stratum corneum*) – **outermost layer**
- the clear layer (*stratum lucidum*)
- the granular layer (*stratum granulosum*)
- the prickle cell layer (*stratum spinosum*)
- the basal cell layer (*stratum germinativum*) – **innermost layer**.

▸ The three outermost layers (horny, clear and granular) consist of dead cells as a result of the process known as keratinisation. The cells in the very outermost layer are dead and scaly and are constantly being rubbed away by friction.
▸ The inner two layers are composed of living cells.
▸ The epidermis does not have a system of blood vessels, therefore all nutrients pass into the cells of the epidermis from blood vessels in the deeper dermis.

The basal cell layer (*stratum germinativum*)

This is the deepest of the five layers. It consists of a single layer of column cells on a basement membrane which separates the epidermis from the dermis. In this layer the new epidermal cells are constantly being reproduced. These cells last about six weeks from reproduction before being discarded into the horny layer. New cells are therefore formed by division, pushing adjacent cells towards the skin's surface. At intervals in the column cells, which divide to reproduce, are the large star-shaped cells called melanocytes which form the pigment melanin, the skin's main colouring agent.

Prickle cell layer (*stratum spinosum*)

This is known as the prickle cell layer because each of the rounded cells contained within it has short projections which make contact with the neighbouring cells and give them a prickly appearance. The living cells of this layer are capable of dividing by the process known as **mitosis**.

Granular layer (*stratum granulosum*)

This layer consists of distinctly shaped cells, containing a number of granules which are involved in the hardening of cells by the process known as **keratinisation**.

Keratinisation refers to the process that cells undergo when they change from living cells with a nucleus to dead cells without a nucleus. This layer links the living cells of the epidermis to the dead cells above.

Clear layer (*stratum lucidum*)

This layer consists of transparent cells which permit light to pass through. It consists of three or four rows of flat, dead cells which are completely filled with keratin; they have no nuclei as the cells have undergone mitosis. The clear layer of the epidermis is thought to form a barrier zone which controls the movement of water through the skin. This layer is very shallow in facial skin, but thick on the soles of the feet and the palms of the hands, and is generally absent in hairy skin.

Horny layer (*stratum corneum*)

This is the most superficial outer layer, consisting of dead, flattened keratinised cells which have taken approximately a month to travel from the basal cell layer. The cells of the horny layer form a waterproof covering for the skin and help to prevent the penetration of bacteria. This outer layer of dead cells is continually being shed; this process is known as **desquamation**.

Cell regeneration

Cell regeneration occurs in the epidermis by the process of mitosis (cell division). It takes approximately a month for a new cell to complete its journey from the basal cell layer, where it is

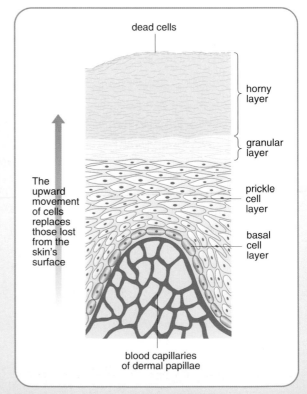

Cell regeneration of the epidermis

reproduced, to the granular layer where it becomes **keratinised**, to the horny layer where it is **desquamated**.

The dermis

The **dermis** lies below the epidermis and is the deeper layer of the skin. Its key functions are to provide nourishment to the epidermis and to give a supporting framework to the tissues.

The dermis has two layers: a superficial papillary layer and a deeper reticular layer.

The superficial papillary layer is made up of fatty connective tissue and is connected to the underside of the epidermis by cone-shaped projections called **dermal papillae** which contain nerve endings and a network of blood and lymphatic capillaries.

The deeper reticular layer is formed of tough fibrous connective tissue which contains the following:

- collagen fibres which help to give the skin strength and resilience
- elastic fibres which help to give the skin elasticity
- reticular fibres which help to support and hold all structures in place.

Cells present in the dermis include:

- mast cells which secrete histamine (involved in allergies), causing dilation of blood vessels to bring blood to the area
- phagocytic cells, which are white blood cells that are able to travel around the dermis, destroying foreign matter and bacteria
- fibroblasts, which are cells that help form new fibrous tissue.

Blood supply

Unlike the epidermis, the dermis has an abundant supply of blood vessels which run through the dermis and the subcutaneous layer.

Arteries carry oxygenated blood to the skin via arterioles and these enter the dermis from below and branch into a network of capillaries around active or growing structures. These **capillary networks** form in the dermal papillae to provide the basal cell layer of the epidermis with food and oxygen. They also surround the sweat glands and *erector pili* muscles, two appendages of the skin.

The capillary networks drain into venules, small veins which carry the deoxygenated blood away from the skin and remove waste products. The dermis is therefore well supplied with capillary blood vessels to bring nutrients and oxygen to the germinating cells in the basal cell layer of the epidermis and to remove waste products from them.

Lymphatic vessels

There are numerous lymphatic vessels in the dermis. They form a network in the dermis facilitating the removal of waste from the skin's tissue. The lymphatic vessels in the skin generally follow the course of veins and are found around the dermal papillae, glands and hair follicles.

Nerves

There is a wide distribution of nerves throughout the dermis. Most nerves in the skin are sensory; they send signals to the brain, and are sensitive to heat, cold, pain, pressure and touch. The dermis also has motor nerves which relay impulses to the brain and are responsible for the dilation and constriction of blood vessels, the secretion of perspiration from the sweat glands and the contraction of the *erector pili* muscles attached to hair follicles.

The subcutaneous layer

This is a thick layer of connective tissue found below the dermis. The types of tissue found in this layer (areolar and adipose) help support delicate structures such as blood vessels and nerve endings.

The subcutaneous layer contains the same collagen and elastin fibres as the dermis and contains the major arteries and veins which supply the skin and form a network throughout the dermis. The fat cells contained within this layer help to insulate the body by reducing heat loss. Below the subcutaneous layer lies the subdermal muscle layer.

Appendages of the skin

The appendages are accessory structures that lie in the dermis of the skin and project onto the surface through the epidermis. These include the hair, the *erector pili* muscles, and the sweat and sebaceous glands.

Hair

Hair is an appendage of the skin which grows from a sac-like depression in the epidermis called a hair follicle. Hair grows all over the body, with the exception of the palms of the hands and the soles of the feet.

The primary function of a hair is physical protection. For example, the hair on the scalp provides partial shading from the sun's rays, and the hairs in the nostrils, eyelashes and eyebrows provide protection from foreign particles.

The structure of a hair

The hair is composed mainly of the protein keratin and is therefore a dead structure.

Longitudinally, the hair is divided into three parts:

- **hair shaft** – the part of the hair that lies above the surface of the skin
- **hair root** – the part of the hair which is found below the skin
- **hair bulb –** the enlarged part at the base of the hair root.

Internally the hair has three layers which all develop from the matrix, which is the active, growing part of the hair:

- **cuticle:** this is the outer layer and is made up of transparent protective scales which overlap one another. The cuticle protects the cortex and gives the hair its elasticity

- **cortex:** this is the middle layer and is made up of tightly packed keratinised cells containing the pigment melanin, which gives the hair its colour. The cortex helps to give strength to the hair
- **medulla:** this is the inner layer and is made up of loosely connected keratinised cells and tiny air spaces. This layer of the hair determines the sheen and colour of the hair because of the reflection of light through the air spaces.

Hair growth

Hair growth originates from the central area of the hair bulb, the matrix, which is the active, growing area where the hair cells divide and reproduce. The living cells produced in the matrix are then pushed upwards from their source of nutrition and are converted to keratin to produce a hair that eventually projects from the open end of the follicle.

The growth cycle of the hair

Hair has a growth pattern which ranges from approximately four to five months for an eyelash hair to approximately four to seven years for a scalp hair.

At the end of each hair's life span, the root of the hair separates from its matrix and remains in the follicle until it falls out or is pulled out. The follicle then shrinks and enters a period of rest. Following its rest period, the follicle will either degenerate completely or enlarge to form a new hair bulb and produce another hair.

Hair colour

Hair colour is determined by the presence of melanin in the cortex and the medulla of the hair shaft. In addition to the standard black colour, the melanocytes in the hair bulb produce two colour variations of melanin: brown and yellow. Blond, light-coloured and red hair have a high proportion of the yellow variant. Brown and black hair possess more of the brown and black melanin.

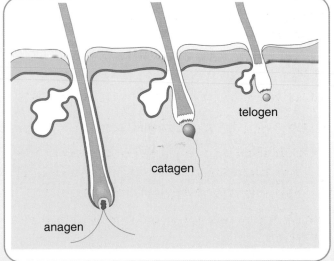

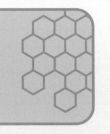

key note

Hair turns grey when the melanocytes in the hair bulb stop producing melanin.

The hair growth cycle

Erector pili muscle

This is a small, smooth muscle which is attached at an angle to the base of a hair follicle, and serves to make the hair stand erect in response to cold.

Sweat glands

There are two types of sweat glands; the majority are called eccrine glands, which are simple, coiled tubular glands that open directly onto the surface of the skin. There are several million of them distributed over the surface of the skin, although they are most numerous on the palms of the hands and the soles of the feet.

Their function is to regulate body temperature and help eliminate waste products. Their active secretion, sweat, is under the control of the sympathetic nervous system.

The other type of sweat glands are called apocrine glands; these are connected with hair follicles and are found only in the genital and underarm regions. They produce a fatty secretion; breakdown of the secretion by bacteria leads to body odour.

Sebaceous glands

These glands are found all over the body, except for the soles of the feet and the palms of the hands. They are more numerous on the scalp, face, chest and back.

Sebaceous glands commonly open into a hair follicle but some open onto the skin surface. They produce an oily substance called sebum which contains fats, cholesterol and cellular debris.

Sebum coats the surface of the skin and the hair shafts, where it prevents excess water loss, lubricates and softens the horny layer of the epidermis and softens the hair.

key note

Indian Head Massage can help to bring about an improvement in a client's skin and hair condition over a period of time. The increased circulation to the skin can increase cell nutrition and regeneration, as well as increase elimination of waste from the skin's tissues. Dead keratinised cells which are blocking the pores of the skin can be loosened by massage and the blood supply can flow more freely to feed the skin and hair with nutrients. Indian Head Massage can also help to increase the production of sebum from the sebaceous glands, helping to lubricate the skin and hair and improve its condition.

activity task

Using the information given in this chapter so far, label the following cross-section diagram of the skin.

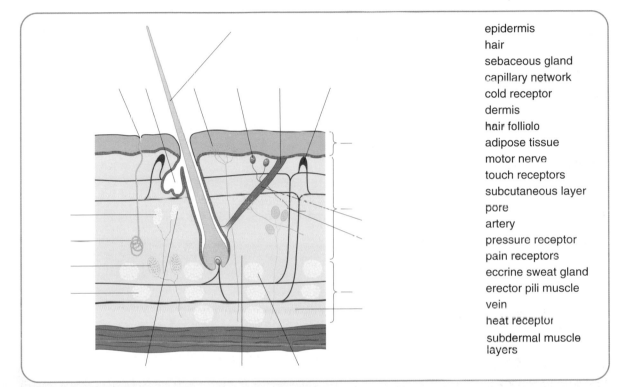

epidermis
hair
sebaceous gland
capillary network
cold receptor
dermis
hair folliolo
adipose tissue
motor nerve
touch receptors
subcutaneous layer
pore
artery
pressure receptor
pain receptors
eccrine sweat gland
erector pili muscle
vein
heat receptor
subdermal muscle layers

Cross-section of the skin

Glossary of useful terms associated with the skin

Allergic reaction

A disorder in which the body becomes hypersensitive to a particular allergen. When irritated by an allergen, the body produces histamine in the skin, as part of the body's defence or immune system.

The effects of different allergens are diverse and they affect different tissues and organs. For instance, certain cosmetics and chemicals can cause rashes and irritation in the skin; certain allergens such as pollen, fur, feathers, mould and dust can cause asthma and hay fever.

If severe, allergies may be extremely serious and result in anaphylactic shock.

Comedone

A collection of sebum, keratinised cells and wastes which accumulates in the entrance of a hair follicle. It may be open or closed. An open comedone is a 'blackhead' contained within the follicle, whereas a closed comedone is a 'whitehead', trapped underneath the skin's surface.

Cyst

An abnormal sac containing liquid or a semi-solid substance. Most cysts are harmless.

Erythema

Reddening of the skin caused by the dilation of blood capillaries just below the epidermis, in the dermis.

Fissure

A crack in the epidermis, exposing the dermis.

Keloid

An overgrowth of an existing scar which grows much larger than the original wound. The surface may be smooth, shiny or ridged. The onset is gradual and is caused by an accumulation or increase in collagen in the immediate area. The colour varies from red, fading to pink and white.

Lesion

A zone of tissue with impaired function, as a result of damage by disease or wounding.

Macule

A small, flat patch of increased pigmentation or discolouration, for example a freckle.

Milia

Sebum trapped in a blind duct with no surface opening. Usually found around the eye area. It appears as pearly, white, hard nodules under the skin.

Mole

Moles are also known as pigmented naevi. They appear as round, smooth lumps on the surface of the skin. They may be flat or raised and vary in size and colour from pink to brown or black. They may have hairs growing out of them.

Naevus

A mass of dilated capillaries. May be pigmented, as in a birthmark.

Papule

Small, raised elevation on the skin, less than 1cm in diameter; may be red in colour. Often develops into a pustule.

Pustule

Small, raised elevation on the skin which contains pus.

Skin tag

Small growth of fibrous tissue, which stands up from the skin and is sometimes pigmented (black or brown).

Scar

A mark left on the skin after a wound has healed. Scars are formed from replacement tissue during the healing of the wound. Depending on the type and extent of damage, the scar may be raised (hypertrophic), rough and pitted (ice pick), or fibrous and lumpy (keloid). Scar tissue may appear smooth and shiny or form a depression in the surface.

Telangiecstasis

This is a term for dilated capillaries, where there is persistent vaso-dilation of capillaries in the skin. Usually caused by extremes of temperature and overstimulation of the tissues, although sensitive and fair skins are more susceptible to this condition.

Tumour

A tumour is formed by an overgrowth of cells; almost every type of cell in the epidermis and dermis is capable of benign or malignant overgrowth. Tumours are lumpy and, even when they cannot be seen, they can be felt underneath the surface of the skin.

Ulcer

A break or open sore in the skin, extending to all its layers.

Vesicles

Small sac-like blisters. A bulla is a vesicle larger than 0.5cm and is commonly called a blister.

Wart

Well-defined benign tumour which varies in size and shape. See viral infections on page 26.

Weal

A raised area of skin, containing fluid, which is white in the centre with a red edge. Is seen in the condition urticaria.

Disorders of the sebaceous gland

Acne vulgaris

A common inflammatory disorder of the sebaceous glands which leads to the overproduction of sebum. It involves the face, back and chest and is characterised by the presence of comedones, papules, and in more severe cases cysts and scars.

Acne vulgaris is primarily androgen-induced and appears most frequently at puberty and usually persists for a considerable period of time.

Rosacea

A chronic inflammatory disease of the face in which the skin appears abnormally red. The condition is gradual and begins with flushing of the cheeks and nose and as the condition progresses it may become pustular. Aggravating factors include hot, spicy foods, hot drinks, alcohol, the menopause, the elements and stress.

Sebaceous cyst

A round, nodular lesion with a smooth, shiny surface, which develops from a sebaceous gland. They are usually found on the face, neck, scalp and back. They are situated in the dermis and vary in size from 5 to 50mm. The cause is unknown.

Seborrhoea

This condition is defined as an excessive secretion of sebum by the sebaceous glands. The glands are enlarged and the skin appears greasy, especially on the nose and the centre zone of the face. The condition may develop into acne vulgaris and is common at puberty, lasting for a few years.

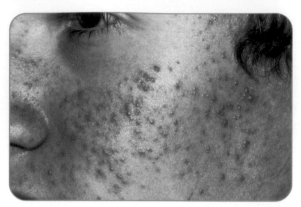
Acne vulgaris

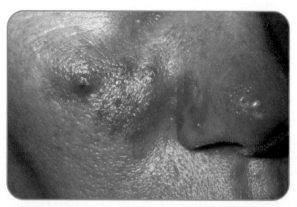
Rosacea

Disorders of the sweat glands

Hyperhidrosis

Excessive production of sweat, affecting the hands, feet and underarms.

Bacterial infections

Boil

A boil begins as a small, inflamed nodule which forms a pocket of bacteria around the base of a hair follicle or a break in the skin. Local injury or lowered constitutional resistance may encourage the development of boils.

Conjunctivitis

This is a bacterial infection following irritation of the conjunctiva of the eye. In this condition the inner eyelid and eyeball appear red and sore and there may be a pus-like discharge from the eye. The infection spreads by contact with the secretions from the eye of the infected person.

Folliculitis

This is a bacterial infection of the hair follicles of the skin and appears as a small pustule at the base of the hair follicle. There is redness, swelling and pain around the hair follicle.

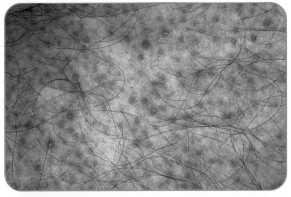

Folliculitis

Sycosis barbae

This is a chronic folliculitis in which there are pustules in the hair follicles and inflammation of the surrounding skin area. Folliculitis is characterised by burning and itching, with pain on manipulation of the hair. Chronic, persistent infection results in spread to the surrounding skin which becomes red and crusted, resembling eczema. The upper lip is particularly susceptible in patients who suffer from chronic nasal discharge from sinusitis or hay fever.

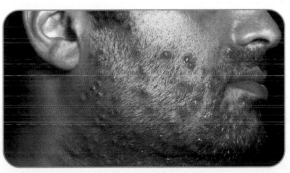

Sycosis barbae

Impetigo

A superficial contagious inflammatory disease caused by streptococcal and staphylococcal bacteria. It is commonly seen on the face and around the ears, and features include weeping blisters which dry to form honey-coloured crusts. (The bacteria are easily transmitted by dirty fingernails and towels.)

Stye

Acute inflammation of a gland at the base of an eyelash, caused by bacterial infection. The gland becomes hard and tender and a pus-filled cyst develops at the centre.

Viral infections of the skin

Herpes simplex (cold sores)

Herpes simplex is normally found on the face and around the lips. It begins as an itching sensation, followed by erythema and a group

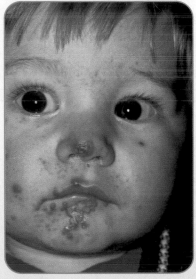

Impetigo

of small blisters which then weep and form crusts. This condition will generally persist for approximately two or three weeks, but will reappear at times of stress, ill health or exposure to sunlight.

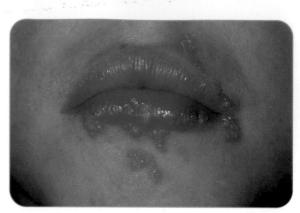
Herpes simplex

Herpes zoster (shingles)

Painful infection along the sensory nerves by the virus that causes chicken pox. Lesions resemble herpes simplex, with erythema and blisters along the lines of the nerves. Areas affected are mostly on the back or upper chest wall. This condition is very painful because of acute inflammation of one or more of the peripheral nerves. Severe pain may persist at the site of shingles for months or even years after the apparent healing of the skin.

Warts

A wart is a benign growth on the skin caused by infection with the human papilloma virus.

* **Plane warts** are smooth in texture with a flat top and are usually found on the face, forehead, the back of the hands and the front of the knees.
* **Plantar warts** or **verrucae** occur on the soles of the feet and are usually the size of a pea.

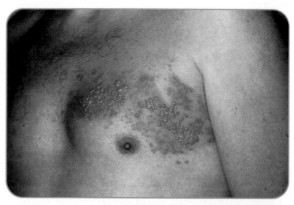
Herpes zoster

Fungal infections of the skin

Ringworm

A fungal infection of the skin which begins as small red papules that gradually increase in size to form a ring. Affected areas on the body vary in severity, from mild scaling to inflamed itchy areas.

Tinea barbae (ringworm of the beard)

Tinea barbae is the name used for fungal infection of the beard and moustache areas. It is less common than tinea capitis and generally affects only adult men.

The skin is usually very inflamed, with red, lumpy areas, pustules

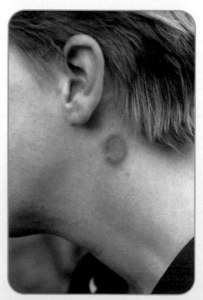
Ringworm

and crusting around the hairs. The hairs can be pulled out easily. Surprisingly, it is not excessively itchy or painful. The cause of tinea barbae is most often an animal fungus, originating from cattle or horses. Tinea barbae most often affects farmers and is caused by direct contact with an infected animal. It is rarely passed from one person to another.

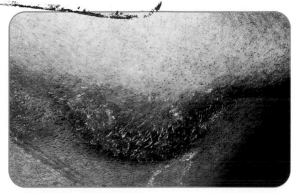

Tinea barbae

Tinea capitis

This is a fungal infection of the scalp (ringworm) and appears as painless, round, hairless patches on the scalp. Itching may be present and the lesion(s) may appear red and scaly.

Tinea pedis (athlete's foot)

This is a highly contagious condition which is easily transmitted in damp, moist conditions such as swimming pools, saunas and showers. Athlete's foot appears as flaking skin between the toes which becomes soft and soggy. The skin may also split and the soles of the feet may occasionally be affected.

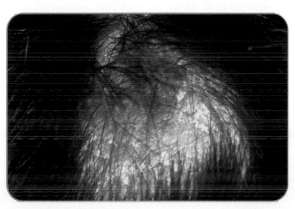

Tinea capitis

Infestation disorders of the skin

Pediculosis (lice)

This condition is commonly known as lice and is a contagious parasitic infection, where the lice live off the blood sucked from the skin.

Head lice are frequently seen in young children and, if not dealt with quickly, may lead to a secondary infection as a result of scratching (impetigo). With head lice, nits may be found in the hair; these are pale grey or brown oval structures found on the hair shaft, close to the scalp. The scalp may appear red and raw because of the patient's scratching.

Body lice are rarely seen. They will occur on an individual with poor personal hygiene and will live and reproduce in seams and fibres of clothing, feeding off the skin. Lesions may appear as papules, scabs, and in severe cases pigmented, dry, scaly skin. Secondary bacterial infection is often present. A client affected by body lice will complain of itching, especially in the shoulder, back and buttock areas.

Scabies

A contagious parasitic skin condition caused by the female mite which burrows into the horny layer of the skin where she lays her eggs. The first noticeable symptom of this condition is severe itching which

worsens at night; papules, pustules and crusted
lesions may also develop.

Common sites for this infestation are the ulnar
borders of the hand, palms of the hands and
between the fingers and toes. Other sites include
the axillary folds, the buttocks, the breasts in the
female and the external genitalia in the male.

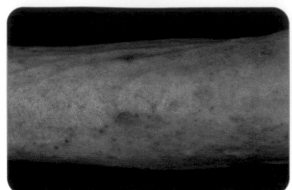

Scabies

Pigmentation disorders

Albinism

A condition in which there is an inherited absence
of pigmentation in the skin, hair and eyes, resulting
in white hair, pink skin and pink eyes. The pink colour is produced by underlying blood vessels which are
normally masked by pigment.

Other clinical signs of this condition include poor eyesight and sensitivity to light.

Chloasma

This is a pigmentation disorder which presents with irregular areas of increased pigmentation, usually on
the face. It commonly occurs during pregnancy, or sometimes the person is affected when taking the
contraceptive pill, because of stimulation of melanin by the female hormone oestrogen.

Lentigo

Also known as 'liver spots'. These are flat, dark patches of pigmentation which are found mainly in the
elderly, on skin exposed to light.

Vitiligo

This condition presents with areas of the skin which
lack pigmentation caused by the basal cell layer of
the epidermis no longer producing melanin. The
cause of vitiligo is unknown.

Naevi

Portwine stain

Also known as a 'deep capillary naevus'. Present at
birth and may vary in colour from pale pink to deep
purple. Has an irregular shape, but is not raised
above the skin's surface. Usually found on the face,
but may also appear on other areas of the body.

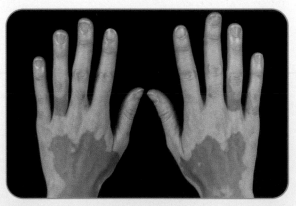

Vitiligo

Spider naevi
A collection of dilated capillaries which radiate from a central papule. Often appear during pregnancy or as the result of 'picking a spot'.

Strawberry mark
Usually develops on a baby before or shortly after birth, but disappears spontaneously before the child reaches the age of ten. It is raised above the skin's surface.

Hypertrophic disorders

Malignant melanoma
A malignant melanoma is a deeply pigmented mole which is life-threatening if it is not recognised and treated promptly. Its main characteristic is a blue–black nodule which increases in size, shape and colour and is most commonly found on the head, neck and trunk. Overexposure to strong sunlight is a major cause and its incidence is increased in young people with fair skins.

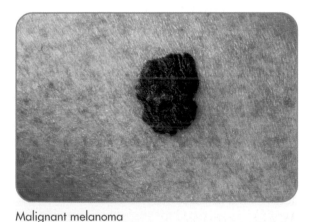

Malignant melanoma

Rodent ulcer
This is a malignant tumour, which starts off as a slow-growing, pearly nodule, often at the site of a previous skin injury. As the nodule enlarges, the centre ulcerates and refuses to heal. The centre becomes depressed and the rolled edges become translucent, revealing many tiny blood vessels. Rodent ulcers do not disappear and if left untreated may invade the underlying bone. **This is the most common form of skin cancer**.

Squamous cell carcinoma
This is a malignant tumour which arises from the prickle cell layer of the epidermis. It is hard and warty and eventually develops a 'heaped up', 'cauliflower' appearance. It is most frequently seen in elderly people.

Inflammatory skin conditions

Contact dermatitis
Dermatitis literally means 'inflammation of the skin'. Contact dermatitis is caused by a primary irritant which causes the skin to become red, dry and inflamed. Substances which are likely to cause this reaction include acids, alkalis, solvents, perfumes, lanolin, detergents and nickels. There may be skin infection as well.

Eczema

A mild to chronic inflammatory skin condition characterised by itchiness, redness and the presence of small blisters that may be dry or weeping if the surface is scratched. Eczema is non-contagious; the cause may be genetic or internal and external influences.

It can cause scaly and thickened skin, mainly at flexures, for example the cubital area of the elbows and the back of the knees.

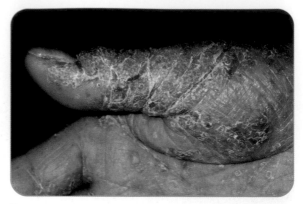

Eczema

Psoriasis

A chronic inflammatory skin condition. Psoriasis may be recognised as the development of well-defined red plaques, varying in size and shape and covered by white or silvery scales. Any area of the body may be affected by psoriasis but the most commonly affected sites are the face, elbows, knees, nails, chest and abdomen. It can also affect joints and the scalp. Psoriasis is aggravated by stress and trauma but is improved by exposure to sunlight.

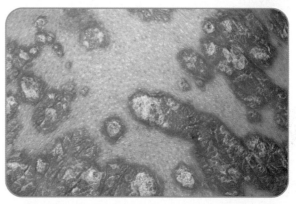

Psoriasis

Seborrhoeic dermatitis

This is a mild to chronic inflammatory disease of hairy areas well supplied with sebaceous glands. Common sites are the scalp, face, axilla and the groin. The skin may appear to have a grey tinge or may be dirty yellow in colour. Clinical signs include slight redness, scaling and dandruff in the eyebrows.

Pityriasis simplex capitis (dandruff)

* **'Dandruff'** is a popular collective name signifying a scaly, flaking scalp condition.
* **Pityriasis simplex capitis** is a non-inflammatory scalp condition which presents as exfoliation of the stratum corneum (outer layer of epidermal cells).

Urticaria

Also known as hives. In this condition, lesions appear rapidly and disappear within minutes or gradually over a number of hours. The clinical signs are development of red weals which may later become white. The area becomes itchy or may sting.

There are a number of causes of urticaria, some of which are an allergic reaction to certain foods, for example strawberries or shellfish, as well as to penicillin, house dust and pet fur. Other causes include stress and sensitivity to light, heat or cold.

activity task

Complete the following table and indicate whether it is possible to offer an Indian Head Massage treatment if a client presents with the following conditions.

Condition	✓ = Treatment possible	✗ = Treatment not possible
Tinea capitis		
Psoriasis		
Pityriasis simplex capitis		
Vitiligo		
Impetigo		
Conjunctivitis		
Rosacea		
Seborrhoeic dermatitis		
Sycosis barbae		

Factors affecting the skin

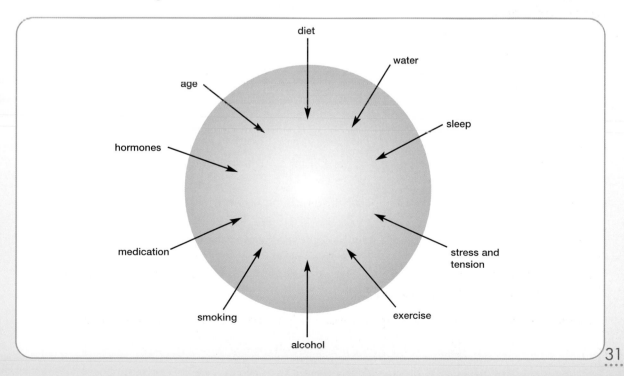

31

- **Diet** – a healthy body is needed for a healthy skin. The skin can be thought of as a barometer of the body's general health.
  ▸ **Vitamin A:** helps repair the body's tissues and helps prevent dryness and ageing
  ▸ **Vitamin B:** helps improve the circulation and the skin's colour, and is essential to cellular oxidation
  ▸ **Vitamin C:** is essential for healing and to maintain levels of collagen in the skin.

- **Water** – drinking an adequate amount of water (approximately six to eight glasses per day) aids the digestive system and helps to prevent a build-up of toxicity in the tissues of the skin.

- **Sleep** – sleep is essential to physical and emotional wellbeing and is one of the most effective regenerators for the skin.

- **Stress and tension** – when the body is subjected to regular stress and tension, these can cause sensitivity and allergies in the skin as well as encourage the formation of lines around the eyes and the mouth.

- **Exercise** – regular exercise promotes good circulation, increased oxygen intake and blood flow to the skin.

- **Alcohol** – alcohol has a dehydrating effect on the skin, and excess consumption causes the blood vessels in the skin to dilate.

- **Smoking** – smoking affects the skin's cells and destroys vitamins B and C which are important for a healthy skin. Smoking dulls the skin by polluting the pores, and increases the formation of lines around the eyes and the mouth.

- **Medication** – medication can affect the skin by causing dehydration or sensitivity and/or allergies.

- **Hormones** – the natural glandular changes of the body have an effect on the condition of the skin throughout life:
  ▸ during **puberty**, the sex hormones stimulate the sebaceous glands, which may cause some imbalance in the skin
  ▸ at the onset of **menstruation**, the skin may erupt because of the adjustment of hormone levels at that time
  ▸ during **pregnancy**, pigmentation changes may occur, but usually disappear after the birth
  ▸ during the **menopause**, the activity of the sebaceous glands is reduced and the skin becomes drier.

- **Age** – the natural process of ageing naturally affects the skin. From the mid-thirties, the skin starts to lose its firmness, and fine lines and wrinkles start to appear. In the forties and fifties, lines and wrinkles will deepen and loss of muscle tone causes sagging of the skin on the cheeks and the neck. The connective tissue in the skin loses its elasticity and becomes less firm, and the skin becomes thinner and finer. As part of the ageing process, the process of cell regeneration in the skin decreases and the skin appears dry and dull.

Factors affecting hair growth

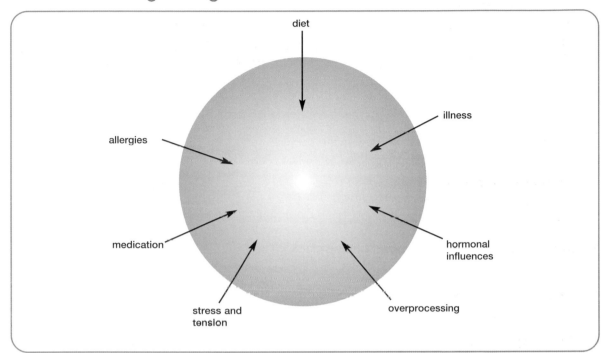

The way our hair looks has a great impact on the way we feel. Shiny, lustrous hair is synonymous with good health and vitality. Factors such as diet, age and hormones directly determine its appearance.

- **Diet** – health of the hair comes from within and therefore a poor diet can affect the condition of the hair. For healthy hair, it is important to have a diet rich in protein, essential fatty acids, and essential vitamins and minerals, such as:
  ‣ Vitamin B complex and vitamin C to help provide nourishment for hair follicles
  ‣ Minerals such as iron, sulphur and zinc, which can help the hair if the important mineral content of the hair is missing and the hair is dull in appearance
  ‣ Vitamin B5, important to help relieve stress in the hair and vitamin A, useful in preventing a dry and scaly scalp.

- **Illness** – prolonged illness and stress can cause both hair loss and greying, because the body is starved of essential nutrients and cell metabolism is slowed down because of infection and/or disease.

- **Hormonal influences** – the hair is often affected by hormonal changes occurring in the body, such as puberty, pregnancy and the menopause. Hair can become more greasy during menstruation. Hair may become dry because of a thyroid problem or there may be a temporary hair loss during pregnancy (especially after delivery). A drop in oestrogen during the menopause can have a profound effect on the hair, causing it to become dry, coarse and brittle.

- **Overprocessing** – perming and dyeing the hair can alter the shaft of the hair, often making it dry and brittle. Frequent use of shampoos full of detergents and chemicals can also dry out the scalp.

- **Stress and tension** – tension in the scalp can reduce the circulation of oxygen and starve the hair root of nutrients needed for healthy growth. Stress can also cause hair loss and premature greying.

- **Medication** – medication can affect the hair by drying the skin, which in turn blocks the follicles with dead, keratinised cells that block the circulation to the scalp.

- **Allergies** – reaction to products used on the hair and scalp may cause sensitisation of the scalp and this can affect the circulation of blood to the hair. Some clients may develop dandruff in response to sensitisation caused by hair products.

The Skeleton

The skeleton is the structure and framework on which other body systems depend for support and protection. It is therefore the physical foundation of the body. The main functions of the skeleton are to provide a means of protection, support and attachment for muscles. The skeleton is very important to a therapist as it provides landmarks for locating muscles.

The areas treated with Indian Head Massage include the upper back, shoulders, neck, upper arms and head, which all have an integral relationship. These parts are discussed in order that the therapist may have a knowledge of the regional anatomy of the treatment area.

Vertebrae of the spine

The spine provides a central axis to the body and consists of 33 individual irregular bones called vertebrae.

The spine is made up of the following:

- 7 cervical vertebrae – bones in the neck
- 12 thoracic vertebrae – bones of the mid-spine
- 5 lumbar vertebrae – bones of the lower back
- 5 sacral vertebrae – fused to form the sacrum
- 4 coccygeal vertebrae – fused to form the coccyx or tail bone.

Vertebrae of the neck

The neck comprises seven bones known as the cervical vertebrae. Although they are the smallest vertebrae in the spine, their bone tissue is denser than those in any other region of the vertebral column.

The top two cervical vertebrae are named C1 and C2.

- **C1** is called the **atlas** and is the bone that sits at the top of the vertebral column embedded in the base of the skull. The atlas supports and balances the head. Sliding joints on either side of the atlas allow the head to move up and down.

THE SPINE

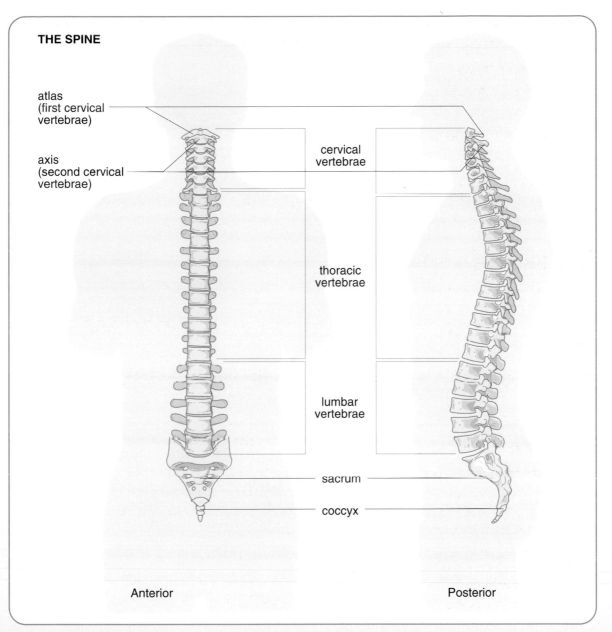

atlas
(first cervical
vertebrae)

axis
(second cervical
vertebrae)

cervical
vertebrae

thoracic
vertebrae

lumbar
vertebrae

sacrum

coccyx

Anterior

Posterior

Vertebrae of the spine

- **C2** is called the **axis** which has a peg-like hook that fits into a notch in the atlas. The ring and peg structure of the atlas and axis allows for movement of the head from side to side.
- The **transverse** processes of the cervical vertebrae are distinctive in that they have transverse foramina (or holes) which serve as passageways for arteries leading to the brain.
- The **spinous** processes of the second through to the fifth cervical vertebrae are uniquely forked to provide attachment for the elaborate lattice of muscles of the neck.

- The **spinous** process of the seventh cervical vertebrae is longer and can be felt through the skin as it protrudes beyond the other cervical spines.

Vertebrae of the mid-spine

There are 12 thoracic vertebrae of the mid-spine and these lie in the thorax where they articulate with the ribs. These vertebrae lie flatter and downwards to allow for attachment of the large muscle groups of the back.

Vertebrae of the lower back

There are five vertebrae that lie in the lower back and they are much larger in size than the vertebrae above them, as they are designed to support body weight.

Sacrum

The sacrum is made up of five fused vertebrae that form a flat, triangular-shaped bone lying in between the pelvic bones.

Coccyx

The coccyx is made up of four coccygeal vertebrae fused together.

The bones of the shoulders

The shoulder girdle connects the upper limbs with the thorax and consists of four bones:

- two clavicles
- two scapulae.

The **clavicle** forms the anterior part of the shoulder girdle. It is a long, slender bone with a double curve which is located at the base of the neck and runs horizontally between the sternum and the shoulders. It articulates with the sternum at its medial end and the scapula at its lateral end. The clavicle acts as a brace for the scapula, helping to hold the shoulders in place.

The **scapulae** form the posterior part of the shoulder girdle and are located on either side of the upper back. The scapula is a large, flat bone, triangular in outline, which articulates with the clavicle and the humerus. The scapula has several prominent processes that serve as attachments for muscles and ligaments. The combined action of scapula, clavicle, humerus and associated muscles allows for a considerable amount of movement of the shoulder and upper limbs.

activity task

Label the bones of the neck and shoulder on the diagram opposite.

Bones of the upper arm

The humerus is the long bone of the upper arm and is the largest bone of the upper extremity. The head of the humerus bone articulates with the scapula to form the shoulder joint and the distal end of the bone joints with the radius and the ulna (bones of the forearm) to form the elbow joint.

Bones of the skull

The skull rests upon the upper end of the vertebral column and weighs around eleven pounds! It consists of 22 bones: eight bones that make up the cranium and 14 forming the facial skeleton.

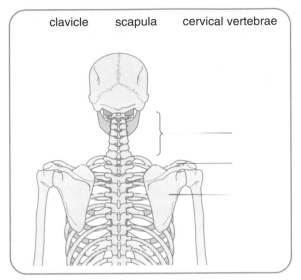

clavicle   scapula   cervical vertebrae

Bones of the neck and shoulder

The cranium encloses and protects the brain and provides a surface attachment for various muscles of the skull. The eight bones of the cranium are as follows:

- one **frontal*** bone forms the anterior part of the roof of the skull, the forehead and the upper part of the orbits or eye sockets
- within the frontal bones are the two frontal sinuses, one above each eye, near the mid-line
- two **parietal*** bones form the upper sides of the skull and the back of the roof of the skull
- two **temporal*** bones form the sides of the skull below the parietal and above and around the ears. The temporal bone contributes to part of the cheekbone via the zygomatic arch (formed by the zygomatic and temporal bones). Located behind the ear and below the line of the temporal bones are the mastoid processes to which the sternomastoid muscles of the neck are attached
- one **sphenoid** bone, which is located in front of the temporal bone and serves as a bridge between the cranium and the facial bones. It articulates with the frontal, temporal, occipital and ethmoid bones
- one **ethmoid** bone which forms part of the wall of the orbit, the roof of the nasal cavity and part of the nasal septum
- the **occipital*** bone which forms the back of the skull.

The bones marked * are considered to be the primary bones of the skull.

key note

There are many openings present in the bones of the skull which act as passages for blood vessels and nerves entering and leaving the cranial cavity. For instance, there is a large opening at the base of the skull called the foramen magnum through which the spinal cord and blood vessels pass to and from the brain.

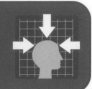

activity task
Label the primary bones of the skull on the diagram below.

The bones of the face

There are 14 facial bones in total and these are mainly in pairs, one on either side of the face:

- **two maxillae*** – these are the largest bones of the face and they form the upper jaw and support the upper teeth. An important part of the maxillae are the maxillary sinuses which open into the nasal cavity
- **one mandible*** – this is the only moveable bone of the skull and forms the lower jaw and supports the lower teeth
- **two zygomatic** – these are the most prominent of the facial bones and they form the cheekbones
- **two nasal** – these small bones form the bridge of the nose
- **two lacrimal** – these are the smallest of the facial bones, and are located close to the medial part of the orbital cavity
- **two turbinate** – these are layers of bone located either side of the outer walls of the nasal cavities
- **one vomer** – this is a single bone at the back of the nasal septum
- **two palatine** – these are L-shaped bones which form the anterior part of the roof of the mouth.

The bones marked ***** are considered to be the primary bones of the face.

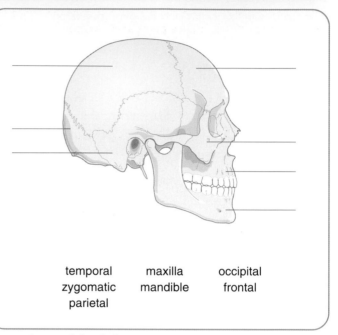

temporal   maxilla   occipital
zygomatic   mandible   frontal
parietal

Primary bones of the skull

The sinuses

There are four pairs of air-containing spaces in the skull and face which are called the sinuses. The function of the sinuses is to lighten the head, provide mucus and act as a resonance chamber for sound. The pairs of sinuses are named according to the facial bones by which they are located. They are the frontal sinuses, the sphenoidal sinuses, the ethomoidal sinuses and the maxillary sinuses (which are the largest).

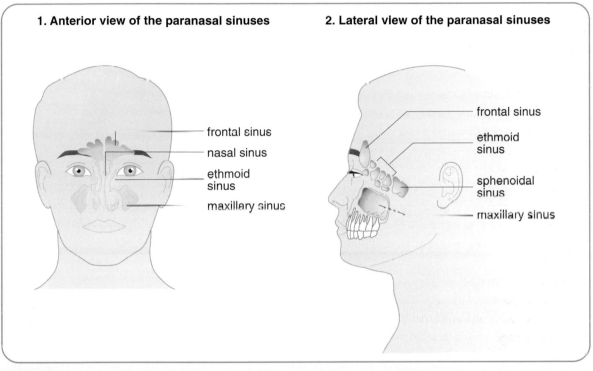

1. Anterior view of the paranasal sinuses

- frontal sinus
- nasal sinus
- ethmoid sinus
- maxillary sinus

2. Lateral view of the paranasal sinuses

- frontal sinus
- ethmoid sinus
- sphenoidal sinus
- maxillary sinus

The sinuses

key note

Indian Head Massage can help to make parts of the skeletal system such as the shoulders and neck more mobile by reducing restrictions in the joints, muscles and their fasciae.

The Muscular System

There are over 600 skeletal or voluntary muscles in the body that collectively help to create body movement, stabilise joints and maintain body posture. Some skeletal muscles lie superficially, while those layered beneath them are known as 'deep' muscles. Detailed on the next page are the main muscles involved in Indian Head Massage.

Muscles of the scalp

Muscle	Position	Attachments	Action	Key Note
Occipitalis	back of the head	to the occipital bone and skin of the scalp	moves the scalp backwards	united to the frontalis muscle by a broad tendon, which covers the skull like a cap
Frontalis	front of the skull and across width of forehead	to the skin of the eyebrows and the frontal bone at the hairline	wrinkles the forehead and raises the eyebrows	used when expressing surprise
Temporalis	at the sides of the skull, above and in front of the ear	to the temporal bone and to the upper part of the mandible	raises the lower jaw when chewing	becomes overtight and painful when there is excessive tension in the jaw

activity task

Label the following muscles relating to the scalp.

frontalis

occipitalis

temporalis

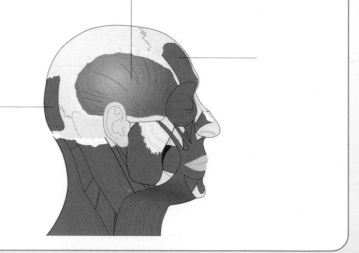

Muscles of the scalp

Muscles of the head and neck

Muscle	Position	Attachments	Action	Key Note
Sterno-mastoid	lies obliquely across each side of the neck	extends from the clavicle and sternum at one end to the mastoid process of the temporal bone (at the back of the ear)	together they flex the neck (pull chin down towards chest); singularly they rotate the head to the opposite side	tends to go into spasm when the head is consistently turned to one side, or pointing downwards, as in working on the telephone and at a desk
Platysma	covers the anterior surface of the neck	extends from chest (upper part of pectoralis major and deltoid) up either side of the neck to the chin	depresses the lower jaw and lower lip	used when yawning and when creating a pouting expression
Orbicularis oculi	circular muscle that surrounds the eye, lying in the subcutaneous tissue of the eyelid	attached to the outer orbits of the eyes, and the skin of the upper and lower eyelids	closes the eye	used when blinking or winking, it also compresses the lacrimal gland, aiding the flow of tears
Orbicularis oris	circular muscle surrounding the mouth	to the maxilla, mandible, lips and the buccinator muscle	closes the mouth	used when shaping the lips for speech and when kissing. It also contracts when tense, as the lips tend to tighten
Corrugator	between the eyebrows	to the frontalis muscle and the inner edge of the eyebrow	brings the eyebrows together	used when frowning

continued over

Muscle	Position	Attachments	Action	Key Note
Procerus	between the eyebrows	to the nasal bones and the frontalis muscle	draws the eyebrows inwards	contraction creates a puzzled expression
Nasalis	sides of the nose	to the maxillae bones and the nostrils	dilates and compresses the nostrils	used when blowing the nose
Zygomatic major and minor	in the cheek region	from the zygomatic bone to the angle of the mouth	draws angle of mouth upwards and laterally	used when laughing
Levator labii superiorus	towards the inner cheek, beside the nose	from upper jaw to the skin at the corners of the mouth and upper lip	raises the upper lip and corner of the mouth	used to create a snarling expression
Risorius	lies horizontally on the cheek, at the corners of the mouth	attaches to the zygomatic bone at one end, and the skin of the corner of the mouth at the other end	pulls corner of mouth sideways and upwards	used to create a grinning expression
Buccinator	main muscle in the cheek	attaches to both upper and lower jaw, from the bones of the jaw to the angle of the mouth	compresses the cheek	used when blowing up a balloon or when using a wind instrument
Mentalis	on the chin	attaches to the lower jaw and the skin of the lower lip	elevates the lower lip and wrinkles skin of chin	used when expressing displeasure and when pouting
Masseter	thick, flattened muscles over the outer part of the cheek and jaw	from the zygomatic arch to the mandible	raises the jaw and exerts pressure on the teeth when chewing	holds a lot of tension and can be felt just in front of the ear when the teeth are clenched

Muscle	Position	Attachments	Action	Key Note
Triangularis	below the corners of the mouth	from the lower jaw to the skin and muscles of the corner of the mouth	draws the corners of the mouth downwards	used to create an expression of sadness

activity task

Label the following muscles of the head and neck.

frontalis   temporalis   orbicularis oris   nasalis
corrugator   zygomatic major   orbicularis oculi   procerus
zygomatic minor   levator labii superious   risorius   buccinator
mentalis   masseter   platysma   triangularis
sternomastoid

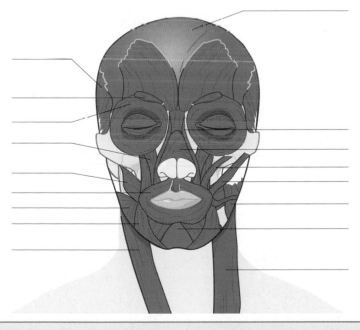

Muscles of the head and neck

Muscles of the back and shoulders

Muscle	Position	Attachments	Action	Key Note
Erector spinae	three bands of muscle that lie in the groove between the vertebral column and the ribs	attaches to the sacrum, iliac crest of pelvis at one end to the ribs, transverse and spinous processes of the vertebrae and the occipital bone at the other end	extension, lateral (side) flexion and rotation of the vertebral column	a very important postural muscle as it helps to extend the spine
Trapezius	large triangular-shaped muscle in the upper back; fibres are arranged in three groups: upper, middle and lower	extends horizontally from the base of the skull, the cervical and thoracic vertebrae to the scapula	upper fibres raise the shoulders; middle fibres pull the scapula towards the spine; lower fibres draw the shoulders downwards	commonly holds a lot of upper body tension, causing discomfort and restrictions in the neck and the shoulders
Levator scapula	long strap-like muscle that runs almost vertically through the neck	from the scapula to the cervical vertebrae of neck	elevates and adducts the scapula (draws the scapula towards spine)	tends to become very tight, which affects the mobility of the neck and the shoulder
Rhomboids	between the scapulae	to the upper thoracic vertebrae at one end and the medial border of the scapula at the other end	adduct the scapula (draw the scapula towards the spine)	often very tight, resulting in aching and soreness in between the scapulae
Supra-spinatus	in the depression above the spine (top ridge) of the scapula	attaches to the spine of the scapula at one end and the humerus at the other end	abducts the humerus (draws the arm away from the body)	often becomes fatigued when working for prolonged periods at a desk or computer, or when driving

Muscle	Position	Attachments	Action	Key Note
Infra-spinatus	below the spine (top ridge) of the scapula	attaches to the middle two-thirds of the scapula at one end and the top of the humerus at the other	rotates the humerus laterally (outwards)	tension in the infraspinatus muscle can affect the range of mobility in the shoulder
Teres major	across the bottom lateral (outer) edge of the scapula	attaches to the bottom lateral (outer) edge of the scapula at one end and the back of the humerus at the other end	adducts and medially (inwardly) rotates humerus	tension in the teres major muscle can restrict the mobility of the shoulder and upper arm
Teres minor	across the lateral edge of the scapula, above teres major	attaches to the lateral (outer) edge of the scapula, above teres major at one end, and into the top of the posterior of the humerus at the other end	rotates humerus laterally (outwards)	tension in the teres minor muscle can restrict the mobility of the shoulder and upper arm

activity task

Label the muscles of the back and shoulders on the diagram on the following page.

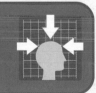

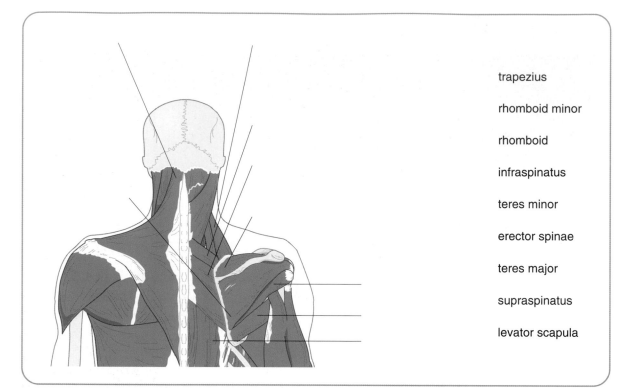

trapezius

rhomboid minor

rhomboid

infraspinatus

teres minor

erector spinae

teres major

supraspinatus

levator scapula

Muscles of the back and shoulders

activity task

Read the following table and then label the muscles of the upper limb.

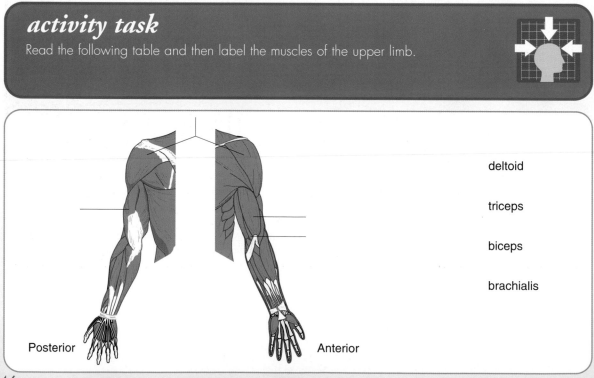

deltoid

triceps

biceps

brachialis

Posterior

Anterior

Muscles of the upper limb

Muscles of the upper limb

Muscle	Position	Attachments	Action	Key Note
Deltoid	caps the top of the humerus and the shoulder	attaches to the clavicle and the spine of the scapula at one end and to the side of the humerus at the other	abducts the arm (draws the arm away from the body), draws the arm backwards and forwards	tends to hold upper body tension and will often go into spasm, along with the trapezius muscle
Biceps	anterior (front) of the upper arm	attaches to the scapula at one end and the radius and flexor muscles of the forearm at the other end	flexes the forearm	becomes tight when the body assumes a tension posture (hunched shoulders and arms, elbows hugged tight against the body)
Triceps	posterior (back) of the humerus	attaches to the posterior of the humerus and the outer edge of the scapula at one end, to the ulna below the elbow at the other end	extension of (straightens) the forearm	becomes tight when the body assumes a tension posture (hunched shoulders and arms, elbows hugged tight against the body)
Brachialis	lies beneath the biceps muscle	attaches to the distal half of the anterior surface of the humerus at one end and the ulna at the other end	flexes the forearm	the most effective flexor muscle of the forearm because of its anatomical position, lying beneath the biceps muscle

Muscles of the chest

Muscle	Position	Attachments	Action	Key Note
Pectoralis major	covers the front of the upper chest	attaches to the clavicle and sternum at one end and to the humerus at the other end	adducts the arm, medially (inwardly), rotates arm	tightness in the pectoralis major muscle may cause constriction of the chest and result in postural distortions (rounded shoulders)
Pectoralis minor	thin strap-like muscle that lies beneath the pectoralis major muscle	from the upper ribs at one end to the scapula at the other end	draws the shoulder downwards and forwards	tightness in the pectoralis minor muscle may cause constriction of the chest and result in postural distortions (rounded shoulders)
Serratus anterior	situated on the side of the chest/rib cage	attaches to the outer surface of the upper eighth or ninth rib at one end to the inner surface of the scapula, along the medial edge nearest the spine	pulls the scapula downwards and forwards	can be affected by chest and breathing difficulties

key note

Muscular tension is often a sign of emotional as well as physical stress.

Indian Head Massage can help to relieve pain from tight, sore muscles as well as relieve muscular fatigue by increasing blood flow, which increases the amount of oxygen and nutrition into the muscles and encourages elimination of waste, absorbing the products of fatigue.

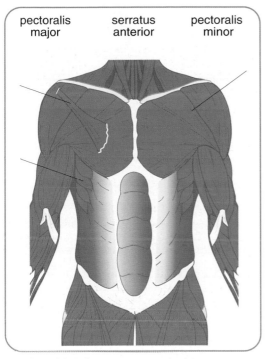

pectoralis major   serratus anterior   pectoralis minor

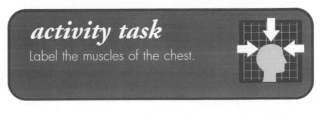

activity task

Label the muscles of the chest.

Muscles of the chest

Posture

Posture is a measure of balance and body alignment, and is the maintenance of strength and tone of the body's muscles against gravity. Good posture is said to occur when the maximum efficiency of the body is maintained with the minimum effort. When evaluating posture, an imaginary line is drawn vertically through the body and this is called the centre of gravity line. From the front or back, this line should divide the body into two symmetrical halves:

- with feet together, the ankles and knees should touch
- the hips should be the same height
- the shoulders should be level
- the sternum and vertebral column should run down the centre of the body, in line with the centre of gravity line
- the head should be erect and not tilted to one side.

Posture varies considerably in individuals and is influenced by factors such as body frame size, heredity, occupation, habits and personality. Additional factors which may also affect posture include clothing, shoes and furniture.

Good posture is important as it:

- allows a full range of movement
- improves physical appearance

- keeps muscle action to a minimum, thereby conserving energy and reducing fatigue
- reduces susceptibility to injuries
- aids the body's systems to function efficiently.

Postural defects

Lordosis

This is an abnormally increased inward curvature of the lumbar spine. In this condition the pelvis tilts forward, and as the back is hollow the abdomen and buttocks protrude, and the knees may be hyperextended. Typical problems associated with this condition are tightening of the back muscles, followed by a weakening of the abdominal muscles. Because of the anterior tilt of the pelvis, hamstring problems are common. Increase in weight or pregnancy may cause or exacerbate this condition.

Kyphosis

This is an abnormally increased outward curvature of the thoracic spine. In this condition the back appears round as the shoulders point forward and the head moves forward. A tightening of the pectoral muscles is common.

Scoliosis

This is a lateral curvature of the vertebral column, which may be to the left or right side. Evident signs of this condition include unequal leg length, distortion of the rib cage, unequal position of the hips or shoulders and curvature of the spine (usually in the thoracic region).

Poor posture may have the following effects on the body:

- produce alterations in body function and movement
- waste energy
- increase fatigue

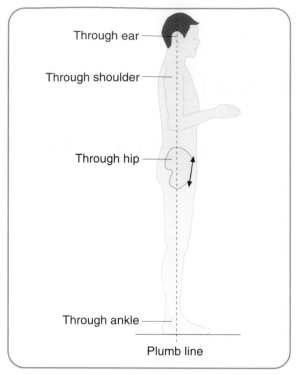
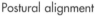

Postural alignment

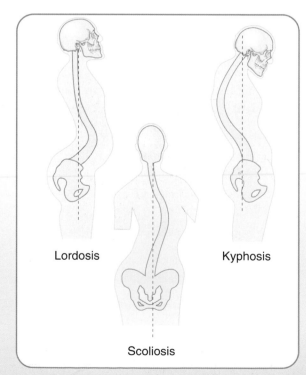

Postural defects

- increase the risk of backache and headaches
- impair breathing
- increase the risk of muscular, ligament or joint injury
- affect circulation
- affect digestion
- give a poor physical appearance.

The Blood Flow to the Head and Neck

The circulatory system comprises blood, the heart and the vast network of circulatory vessels known as arteries, veins and capillaries. The primary function of the circulatory system is transportation. Within the cardiovascular system there are two circuits: the pulmonary circulation and the systemic circulation.

The pulmonary circulation brings deoxygenated blood from the right ventricle of the heart to the alveoli of the lungs to release carbon dioxide and to regain oxygen. Oxygenated blood returns to the left atrium of the heart and moves into the systemic circuit with the contraction of the left ventricle.

The systemic circuit carries oxygenated blood around the body via the body's main artery, the aorta.

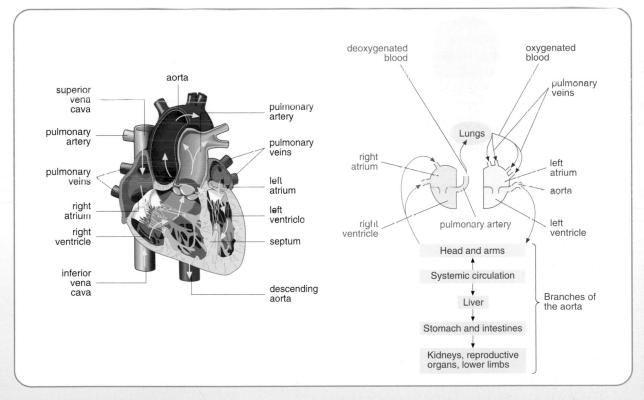

Blood circulation and the heart

On leaving the left ventricle, the aorta emerges from the top of the heart. It passes superiorly for a short distance as the ascending aorta and curves to form the arch of the aorta before it passes inferiorly as the descending aorta. As the aorta emerges from the heart, it subdivides to form the main trunk called the **brachiocephalic trunk**, which splits and forms the **common carotid artery**, which supplies oxygenated blood to the head, face and neck and the **subclavian artery**, which supplies blood to the shoulders, chest wall, arms, back and central nervous system.

Arterial blood supply to the head and neck

Blood is supplied to parts within the neck, head and brain through branches of the subclavian and common carotid arteries.

The **common carotid artery** extends from the brachiocephalic trunk and extends on each side of the neck and divides at the level of the larynx into two branches:

- the **internal** carotid artery
- the **external** carotid artery.

The **internal carotid artery** passes through the temporal bone of the skull to supply oxygenated blood to the brain, eyes, forehead and part of the nose.

The **external carotid artery** is divided into branches (facial, temporal and occipital arteries) which supply the skin and muscles of the face, side and back of the head respectively. This vessel also supplies more superficial structures of the head and neck; these include the salivary glands, scalp, teeth, nose, throat, tongue and thyroid gland.

The **vertebral arteries** are a main division of the subclavian artery. They arise from the subclavian arteries in the base of the neck, near the tip of the lungs. They pass upwards through the openings (foramina) of transverse processes of the cervical vertebrae and unite to form a single basilar artery. The basilar artery then terminates by dividing into two posterior cerebral arteries that supply the occipital and temporal lobes of the cerebrum.

activity task

Using the information given opposite, label the main blood vessels supplying oxygenated blood to the head and neck on the diagram below.

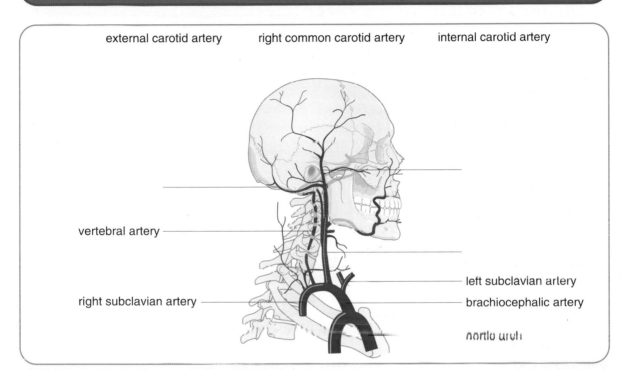

external carotid artery   right common carotid artery   internal carotid artery

vertebral artery

right subclavian artery

left subclavian artery

brachiocephalic artery

aortic arch

Blood vessels of the head and neck (carotid arteries)

Venous drainage from the head and neck

The majority of blood draining from the head is passed into three pairs of veins: the external jugular veins, the internal jugular veins and the vertebral veins. Within the brain, all veins lead to the internal jugular veins.

The **external** jugular vein is smaller than the internal jugular and lies superficial to it. It receives blood from superficial regions of the face, scalp and neck. The external jugular veins descend on either side of the neck, passing over the sternomastoid muscles and beneath the platysma. They empty into the right and left subclavian veins in the base of the neck.

The **internal** jugular vein forms the major venous drainage of the head and neck and is a deep vein that parallels the common carotid artery. It collects deoxygenated blood from the brain and passes downwards through the neck beside the common carotid arteries to join the subclavian veins.

The **vertebral veins** – these descend from the transverse openings (or foramina) of the cervical vertebrae and enter the subclavian veins. The vertebral veins drain deep structures of the neck such as the vertebrae and muscles.

activity task

Using the information given, label the main blood vessels draining deoxygenated
blood from the head and neck on the diagram below.

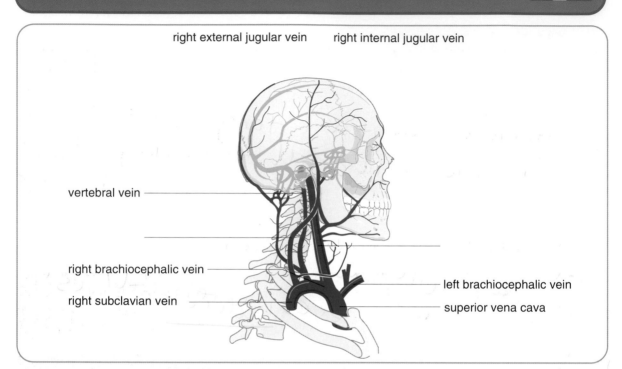

right external jugular vein   right internal jugular vein

vertebral vein

right brachiocephalic vein

right subclavian vein

left brachiocephalic vein

superior vena cava

Blood vessels of the head and neck (jugular veins)

key note

Indian Head Massage can help to enhance the circulation of blood and hence
increase cell nutrition and elimination of cellular waste to and from the head and neck.
The improved circulation to the head also helps to refresh the brain, relieving stress,
tension and fatigue.

The Lymphatic System

The lymphatic system is a one-way drainage system that removes excess fluid from the body's tissues and
returns it to the circulatory system. It is also important in helping the body to fight infection.

Lymphatic vessels form a network of tubes that extend all over the body. The smallest of the vessels –
lymphatic capillaries – end blindly in the body's tissues. Here they collect a liquid called lymph which
leaks out of the body capillaries and accumulates in the tissues. Once collected, lymph flows in one
direction along progressively larger lymphatic vessels. Along the network of lymphatic vessels are lymph

nodes which filter bacteria and micro-organisms from the lymph as it passes through them. The cleansed lymph is then collected by two main lymphatic ducts (the thoracic and the right lymphatic ducts) which empty the lymph into the bloodstream.

The lymphatic system therefore returns the excess fluid which accumulates in the body's tissues back into the bloodstream, while at the same time filtering micro-organisms and releasing antibodies to help the body to fight infection.

key note

The movement of lymph throughout the lymphatic system is known as lymphatic drainage and it begins in the lymphatic capillaries. The movement of lymph out of the tissue spaces and into the lymphatic capillaries is assisted by the pressure exerted by the compression of skeletal muscles. This explains why techniques such as Indian Head Massage are an effective way of draining lymph.

Lymphatic drainage of the head and neck

The main groups of lymphatic nodes relating to the head and neck are:

Name of lymph nodes	Position	Areas lymph is drained from
Cervical (deep)	deep within the neck, located along the path of the larger blood vessels (carotid artery and internal jugular vein)	drains lymph from the larynx, oesophagus, posterior of the scalp and neck, superficial part of chest and arm
Cervical (superficial)	located at the side of the neck, over the sternomastoid muscle	drains lymph from the lower part of the ear and the cheek region
Submandibular	beneath the mandible	drains chin, lips, nose, cheeks and tongue
Occipital	at the base of the skull	drains back of scalp and the upper part of the neck
Mastoid (Post auricular)	behind the ear in the region of the mastoid process	drains the skin of the ear and the temporal region of the scalp
Parotid	at the angle of the jaw	drains nose, eyelids and ear

activity task

Using the information given, label the main lymphatic nodes relating to the head and neck on the diagram below.

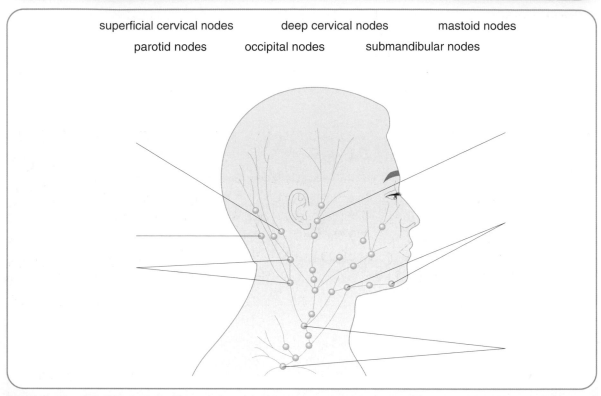

superficial cervical nodes   deep cervical nodes   mastoid nodes

parotid nodes   occipital nodes   submandibular nodes

Lymph nodes of the head and neck

- The right side of the head, neck and right arm drain into the right lymphatic duct and then into the right subclavian vein.
- The left side of the head, neck, the left arm (as well as the lower limbs and abdomen) drain into the left subclavian vein.

The Nervous System

The nervous system comprises the brain, spinal cord and nerves (neurones) which together form a communication network to co-ordinate the various actions of the body. The nervous system works on the same principle as a computer in that it receives information, processes the information and produces an output. The information received reaches the brain from the sensory organs and internal organs; the information is then processed within the brain. The output is through the action of organs, muscles or glands.

The nervous system contains billions of interconnecting neurones which are designed to transmit nerve impulses. There are three types of neurones:

- **sensory neurones**: receive stimuli from sensory organs and receptors and transmit the impulse to the spinal cord and brain. Sensations transmitted by sensory neurones include heat, cold, pain, taste, smell, sight and hearing
- **motor neurones**: conduct impulses away from the brain and the spinal cord to muscles and glands to stimulate them into carrying out their activities
- **association (mixed) neurones**: these link sensory and motor neurones, helping to form the complex pathways that enable the brain to interpret incoming sensory messages and decide on what should be done, and send out instructions in response along motor pathways to keep the body functioning properly.

key note

It is important for therapists to have a basic knowledge of the nervous system to understand its effects in relation to Indian Head Massage, of inducing relaxation and minimising pain. Clients will experience the effects of massage on their muscle tension via the sensory nerves in their muscles. Techniques used in Indian Head Massage help the client to become aware of specific areas of tension and can thereby initiate relaxation and reduce the unconscious motor message (of tension) to the muscles.

The nervous system has two main parts:

- the **central** nervous system (the main control system) that consists of the **brain** and the **spinal cord**
- the **peripheral** nervous system consisting of 31 pairs of **spinal nerves**, 12 pairs of **cranial nerves** and the **autonomic nervous system**.

The central nervous system

The brain

The brain is an extremely complex mass of nervous tissue lying within the skull. It is the main communication centre of the nervous system and its function is to co-ordinate the nerve stimuli received and effect the correct responses. The main parts of the brain include the following:

The cerebrum – this is the largest portion of the brain and makes up the front and top part of the brain. It is divided into two large cerebral hemispheres. The outer layer of the cerebrum is called the cerebral cortex and is the region where the main functions of the cerebrum are carried out. The cortex is concerned with all forms of conscious activity: sensations such as vision, touch, hearing, taste and smell; control of voluntary movements; reasoning; emotion; and memory.

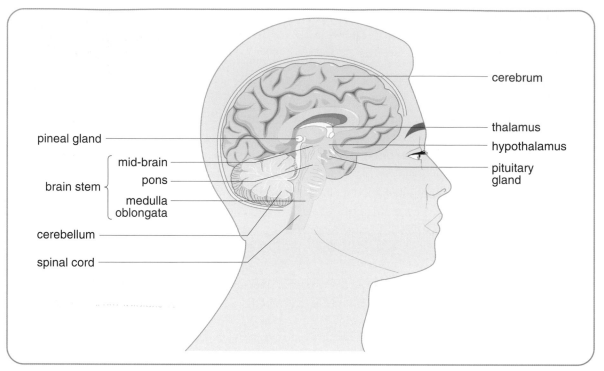

The brain

The cortex of each cerebral hemisphere has a number of functional areas:

* **sensory areas** – these receive impulses from sensory organs all over the body; there are separate sensory areas for vision, hearing, touch, taste and smell
* **motor areas** – these areas have motor connections through motor nerve fibres with voluntary muscles all over the body
* **association areas** – in these areas association takes place between information from the sensory areas and remembered information from past experiences. Conscious thought then takes place and decisions are made which often result in conscious motor activity controlled by motor areas.

The brain requires a continuous supply of glucose and oxygen as it is unable to store glycogen, unlike the liver and muscles.

The thalamus
This is a relay and interpretation centre for all sensory impulses, except olfaction.

The hypothalamus
This small structure governs many important homeostatic functions. It regulates the autonomic nervous system and the endocrine by governing the pituitary gland. It controls hunger, thirst, temperature regulation, anger, aggression, hormones, sexual behaviour, sleep patterns and consciousness.

The pituitary gland

This is a pea-shaped body attached beneath the hypothalamus in a bony cavity at the base of the skull. It is known as the master endocrine gland as its hormones control and stimulate other glands to produce their hormones.

The pineal gland

This is a pea-sized mass of nerve tissue attached by a stalk in the central part of the brain. It is located deep between the cerebral hemispheres, where it is attached to the upper portion of the thalamus.

The pineal gland secretes a hormone called melatonin, which is involved in the regulation of circadian rhythms, patterns of repeated activity that are associated with the environmental cycles of day and night, such as sleep/wake rhythms. The pineal gland is also thought to influence the mood.

The cerebellum

The cerebellum is a cauliflower-shaped structure located at the posterior of the cranium, below the cerebrum. The cerebellum is concerned with muscle tone, the co-ordination of skeletal muscles and balance.

The brain stem contains three main structures:

- the **mid-brain** – this contains the main nerve pathways connecting the cerebrum and the lower nervous system as well as certain visual and auditory reflexes that co-ordinate head and eye movements with things seen and heard
- the **pons** – this is below the mid-brain and relays messages from the cerebral cortex to the spinal cord
- the **medulla oblongata** – this is often considered the most vital part of the brain. It is an enlarged continuation of the spinal cord and connects the brain with the spinal cord. Control centres within the medulla oblongata include those for the heart, lungs and intestines.

The spinal cord

The spinal cord is an extension of the brain stem which extends from an opening at the base of the skull down to the second lumbar vertebra. Its function is to relay impulses to and from the brain. Sensory tracts conduct impulses to the brain and motor tracts conduct impulses from the brain.

> ### key note
>
> Within the spinal cord there are two pathways for sensory information to reach the brain:
>
> - the **fast** pathway that transmits impulses rapidly relates to receptors sensitive to light pressure, vibration and touch
>
> - the **slow** pathway transmits information about pain, temperature and pressure.
>
> When the fast pathway is activated (ie through massage to the skin), the pain pathway is inhibited, as pleasant sensations from the massage arrive at the brain before the pain sensation, thereby helping to displace the awareness of pain.

The peripheral nervous system

This is the communication pathway connecting the central nervous system to the rest of the body.

It consists of:

- **31 pairs of spinal nerves**

  The spinal nerves pass out of the spinal cord and each has two thin branches which link it with the autonomic nervous system. Spinal nerves receive sensory impulses from the body and transmit motor signals to specific regions of the body, thereby providing two-way communication between the central nervous system and the body.

  Each of the spinal nerves is numbered and named according to the level of the spinal column from which it emerges. There are:

  ▸ eight cervical
  ▸ twelve thoracic
  ▸ five lumbar
  ▸ five sacral
  ▸ one coccygeal.

  Each spinal nerve is divided into several branches, forming a network of nerves or plexuses which supply different parts of the body:

  ▸ the **cervical plexuses** of the neck supply the skin and muscles of the head, neck and upper region of the shoulders
  ▸ the **brachial plexuses** supply the skin and muscles of the arm, shoulder and upper chest
  ▸ the **lumbar plexuses** supply the front and sides of the abdominal wall and part of the thigh
  ▸ the **sacral plexuses** at the base of the abdomen supply the skin, muscles and organs of the pelvis
  ▸ the **coccygeal plexus** supplies the skin in the area of the coccyx and the muscles of the pelvic floor.

- **12 pairs of cranial nerves**

  The cranial nerves lead to and from the brain and control feeling and function of the various parts of the head and face, including the muscles, eyes, ears and nose. Some of the nerves are mixed, containing both motor and sensory nerves, while others are either sensory or motor.

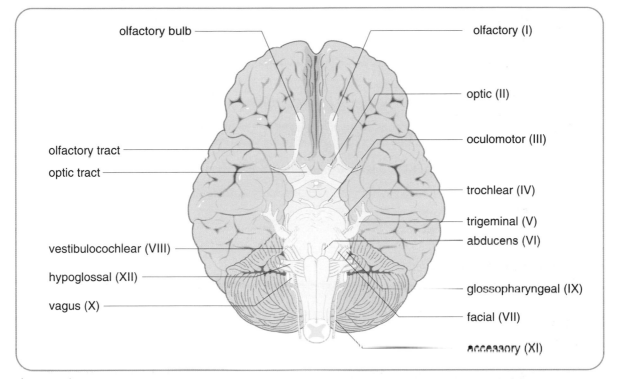

The cranial nerves

▸ **I – olfactory nerve**

This is a sensory nerve of olfaction (smell).

▸ **II – optic nerve**

This is a sensory nerve of vision.

▸ **III – oculomotor nerve**

This is a mixed nerve that innervates both internal and external muscles of the eye and a muscle of the upper eyelid.

▸ **IV – trochlear nerve**

This is the smallest of the cranial nerves and is a motor nerve that innervates the superior oblique muscle of the eyeball that helps you look upwards.

▸ **V – trigeminal nerve**

This is a mixed nerve (containing motor and sensory nerves) that conducts impulses to and from several areas in the face and neck. It also controls the muscles of mastication (the masseter, the temporalis and the pterygoids). It has three main branches – ophthalmic branch, maxillary branch and mandibular branch:

- the **opthalmic** branch carries sensations from the eye, nasal cavity, skin of forehead, upper eyelid, eyebrow and part of the nose
- the **maxillary** branch carries sensations from the lower eyelid, upper lip, gums, teeth, cheek, nose, palate and part of the pharynx
- the **mandibular** branch carries sensations from the lower gums, teeth, lips, palate and part of the tongue.

▸ **VI – abducens**

This is a mixed nerve that innervates only the lateral rectus muscle of the eye, which helps you look to the side.

▸ **VII – facial**

This is a mixed nerve that conducts impulses to and from several areas in the face and neck. The sensory branches are associated with the taste receptors on the tongue and the motor fibres transmit impulses to the muscles of facial expression.

▸ **VIII – vestibulocochlear**

This is a sensory nerve that transmits impulses generated by auditory stimuli and stimuli related to equilibrium, balance and movement.

▸ **IX – glossopharyngeal**

This is a mixed nerve that innervates structures in the mouth and throat. It supplies motor fibres to part of the pharynx and to the parotid salivary glands and sensory fibres to the posterior third of the tongue and the soft palate.

▸ **X – vagus**

This is unlike the other cranial nerves in that it has branches to numerous organs in the thorax and abdomen as well as the neck. It supplies motor nerve fibres to the muscles of swallowing and motor nerve fibres to the heart and organs of the chest cavity. Sensory fibres carry impulses from the organs of the abdominal cavity and the sensation of taste from the mouth.

▸ **XI – accessory**

This functions primarily as a motor nerve, innervating muscles in the neck and upper back (such as the trapezius and the sternomastoid), as well as muscles of the palate, pharynx and larynx.

▸ **XII – hypoglossal**

This is a motor nerve that innervates the muscles of the tongue.

The autonomic nervous system

This is the part of the nervous system that controls the automatic body activities of smooth and cardiac muscle and the activities of glands. It is divided into the sympathetic and parasympathetic divisions, which possess complementary responses.

The activity of the sympathetic system is to prepare the body for expending energy and dealing with emergency situations.

Its effects include:

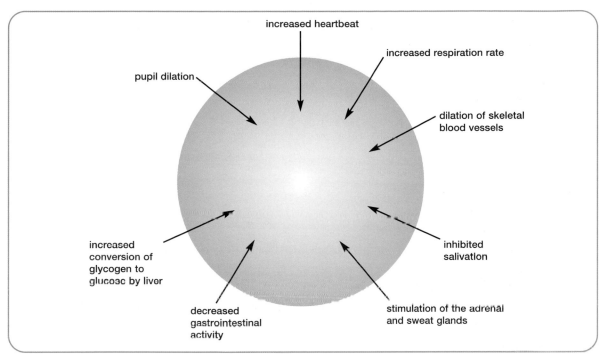

increased heartbeat

increased respiration rate

pupil dilation

dilation of skeletal blood vessels

increased conversion of glycogen to glucose by liver

inhibited salivation

decreased gastrointestinal activity

stimulation of the adrenal and sweat glands

The parasympathetic nervous system balances the action of the sympathetic division by working to conserve energy and create the conditions needed for rest and sleep.

Effects of the **parasympathetic activity** include:

* resting heart rate
* resting respiratory rate
* constriction of skeletal blood vessels
* increased gastrointestinal activity
* pupil constriction
* stimulated salivation.

key note

The sympathetic nervous system is activated at times of anger, fright, anxiety or any type of emotional upset, whether real or imagined. The relaxing effects of an Indian Head Massage can help to *decrease* the effects of the sympathetic nervous system, while *stimulating* parasympathetic activity to promote relaxation and reduce stress levels. It can also help to reduce stress hormones, such as cortisol, by activating the relaxation process. Indian Head Massage is also thought to increase serotonin levels which can help to decrease stress levels and depression.

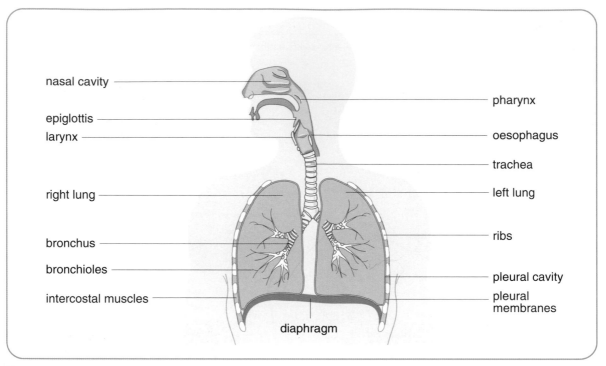

The respiratory tract

Respiration

Oxygen is needed by every cell of the body for survival and delivery; respiration is the process by which the living cells of the body receive a constant supply of oxygen and remove carbon dioxide and other gases. The respiratory system consists of the nose, the pharynx, the larynx, the trachea, the bronchi and the lungs, which provide the passageway for air in and out of the body.

During inhalation, air is drawn in through the nose, pharynx, trachea and bronchi and into the lungs. Inside the lungs, each bronchus divides to form a tree of tubes called bronchioles which progressively increase in diameter and end in microscopic air sacs called alveoli. Oxygen from the air that reaches the alveoli diffuses through the alveolar walls and into the surrounding blood capillaries. This oxygen-rich blood is carried first to the heart and is then pumped to cells throughout the body. Carbon dioxide diffuses out of the blood into the alveoli and is removed from the body during exhalation.

The mechanism of respiration

The mechanism of respiration is the means by which air is drawn in and out of the lungs and is an active process where the muscles of respiration contract to increase the volume of the thoracic cavity.

The major muscle of respiration is the diaphragm. During inspiration the diaphragm contracts and flattens, increasing the volume of the thoracic cavity, and is responsible for 75 per cent of air movement into the

Rib movements in breathing

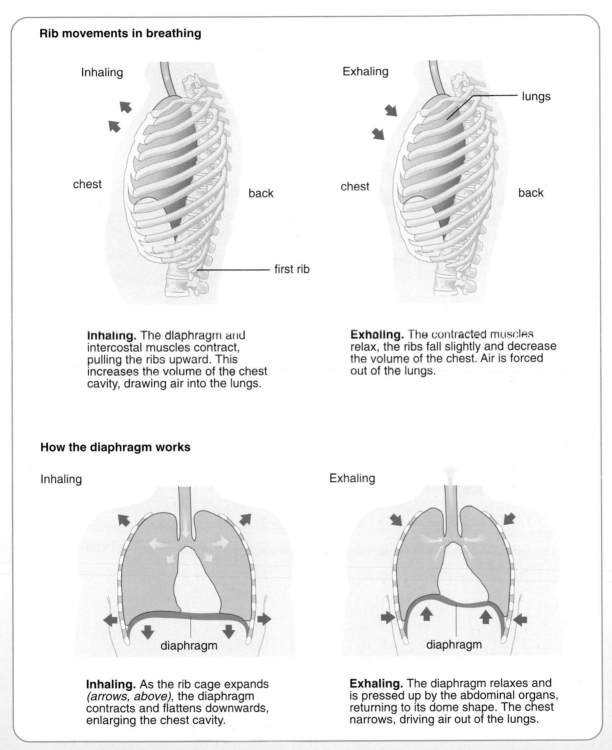

Inhaling

chest   back

first rib

Exhaling

lungs

chest   back

Inhaling. The diaphragm and intercostal muscles contract, pulling the ribs upward. This increases the volume of the chest cavity, drawing air into the lungs.

Exhaling. The contracted muscles relax, the ribs fall slightly and decrease the volume of the chest. Air is forced out of the lungs.

How the diaphragm works

Inhaling

diaphragm

Exhaling

diaphragm

Inhaling. As the rib cage expands *(arrows, above)*, the diaphragm contracts and flattens downwards, enlarging the chest cavity.

Exhaling. The diaphragm relaxes and is pressed up by the abdominal organs, returning to its dome shape. The chest narrows, driving air out of the lungs.

The mechanism of respiration

lungs. The external intercostals are also involved in respiration and upon contraction they increase the depth of the thoracic cavity by pulling the ribs upwards and outwards.

The external intercostal muscles are responsible for bringing approximately 25 per cent of the volume of air into the lungs.

The combined contraction of the diaphragm and the external intercostals increases the thoracic cavity, which then decreases the pressure inside the thorax so that air from outside the body enters the lungs. Other accessory muscles which assist in inspiration include the sternomastoid, serratus anterior, pectoralis minor, pectoralis major and the scalene muscles in the neck.

During normal respiration the process of expiration is passive and is brought about by the relaxation of the diaphragm and the external intercostal muscles. This increases the internal pressure inside the thorax so that air is pushed out of the lungs. In forced expiration, the process of expiration becomes active and is assisted by muscles such as the internal intercostals which help to depress the ribs. Abdominal muscles such as the external and internal obliques, rectus abdominus and the transversus abdominus help to compress the abdomen and force the diaphragm upwards, thus assisting expiration.

key note

Breathing affects both our physiological and psychological state. By freeing tight respiratory muscles, Indian Head Massage can help to increase the vital capacity and function of the lungs.

SELF-ASSESSMENT QUESTIONS

1 *In which layer of the epidermis does keratinisation occur?*

  a *horny layer*

  b *granular layer*

  c *clear layer*

  d *basal cell layer.*

2 *Which is the thinnest layer of the skin?*

  a *dermis*

  b *epidermis*

  c *subcutaneous layer*

  d *subdermal layer.*

SELF-ASSESSMENT QUESTIONS

3 Hair growth occurs from the

   a cuticle

   b cortex

   c medulla

   d matrix.

4 Hair grows from a sac-like depression called the

   a hair shaft

   b hair root

   c hair follicle

   d hair bulb.

5 The sebaceous glands produce an oily substance called

   a sweat

   b lactic acid

   c sebum

   d keratin

6 Which layer lies beneath the subcutaneous layer?

   a papillary layer

   b reticular layer

   c clear layer

   d subdermal muscle layer.

7 Which of the following is NOT a function of the skin?

   a protection

   b heat regulation

   c fight infection

   d absorption.

SELF-ASSESSMENT QUESTIONS

8 How many bones are located in the neck?

a 8

b 10

c 12

d 7.

9 A bone of the skull that forms the sides of the skull above and around the ears is called the

a frontal bone

b temporal bone

c occipital bone

d ethmoid bone.

10 A bone of the face that forms the lower jaw is called the

a maxilla

b zygomatic

c mandible

d lacrimal.

11 The muscle that extends from the chest, up the sides of the neck to the chin is called the

a pectoralis major

b occipitalis

c temporalis

d platsyma.

12 The fan-shaped muscle on the side of the skull, above and in front of the ear, is called the

a occipitalis

b buccinator

c mentalis

d temporalis.

SELF-ASSESSMENT QUESTIONS

13 The muscle that surrounds the eye is called

    a orbicularis oris

    b risorius

    c masseter

    d orbicularis oculi.

14 The action of the risorius muscle is to

    a raise the corner of the mouth

    b close the mouth

    c draw and corners of the mouth laterally

    d elevate the lower lip.

15 The action of the sternomastoid muscle is to

    a depress the mandible

    b extend the head

    c elevate and retract the lower jaw

    d turn the head to one side.

16 The action of the buccinator muscle is to

    a raise the lower jaw

    b compress the cheek

    c elevate and retract the lower jaw

    d elevate the lower lip.

17 The name of the blood vessels that are responsible for supplying oxygenated blood to the head and neck is

    a the brachiocephalic arteries

    b the subclavian arteries

    c the jugular veins

    d the carotid arteries.

SELF-ASSESSMENT QUESTIONS

18 The name of the blood vessels responsible for draining deoxygenated blood from the head and neck is

a the vertebral veins

b the superior vena cava

c the brachiocephalic veins

d the jugular veins.

19 The lymph nodes that drain lymph from the back of the scalp and the upper part of the neck are called

a submandibular nodes

b deep cervical nodes

c occipital nodes

d parotid nodes.

20 The lymph nodes that drain lymph from the larynx, oesophagus, posterior of the scalp and neck, superficial part of the chest and arm are called

a superficial cervical nodes

b mastoid nodes

c deep cervical nodes

d occipital nodes.

21 The central nervous system consists of

a the sympathetic and parasympathetic nervous systems

b the facial and spinal nerves

c the brain and the spinal cord

d the autonomic nervous system.

22 Which branches of nerves (plexuses) supply the skin and muscles of the head, neck and upper region of the shoulders?

a cervical plexuses

b brachial plexuses

c lumbar plexuses

d sacral plexuses.

SELF-ASSESSMENT QUESTIONS

23 Which of the following cranial nerves controls the muscles of mastication?

a facial

b vestibulocochlear

c vagus

d trigeminal.

24 Which of the following is NOT an effect of the sympathetic nervous system?

a pupil dilation

b increased gastrointestinal activity

c dilation of skeletal blood vessels

d increased heartbeat.

25 The process of inspiration is brought about by

a the combined relaxation of the diaphragm and the internal intercostal muscles

b the combined contraction of the diaphragm and the external intercostal muscles

c the combined relaxation of the diaphragm and the external intercostal muscles

d the combined contraction of the diaphragm and the internal intercostal muscles.

Conditions Affecting the Head, Neck and Shoulders

3

A considerable increase in stress levels in sophisticated present-day life has led to a great deal of interest in holistic therapies such as Indian Head Massage, which continues to grow in popularity. More and more people are seeking the benefits of an Indian Head Massage treatment to help improve their emotional and physical wellbeing.

Therapists practising Indian Head Massage need to be knowledgeable within the sphere of their chosen therapy, but also be sufficiently familiar with conditions affecting the head, neck and shoulders in order to design a safe and effective treatment plan that is adapted to the client's needs.

By the end of this chapter, you will be able to relate the following to your practical work:

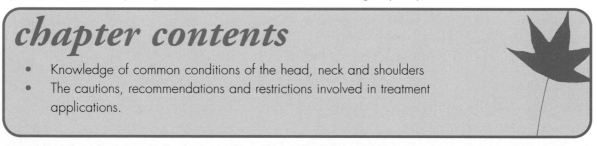

chapter contents

- Knowledge of common conditions of the head, neck and shoulders
- The cautions, recommendations and restrictions involved in treatment applications.

This knowledge will help to empower therapists to make an informed decision as to a suitable treatment plan that is within safe and ethical medical guidelines. It is very important that a therapist never diagnoses a client's medical condition, and refers the client to their GP before any form of treatment is commenced.

key note

It should be noted that while the information given reflects an accurate representation of the condition in generic terms, all clients will vary in the severity of their condition. Each client should be individually assessed as to their condition at the time of the proposed treatment and re-assessed on subsequent treatments. The guidelines given are meant as a general guide and thus therapists are encouraged to seek further clarification of a client's medical condition from the GP and from the client themselves.

Alopecia

A term used to describe temporary baldness or severe hair loss which may follow illness, shock, a period of extreme stress, or may be the side-effect of drug therapy (e.g. chemotherapy). It is important to distinguish temporary baldness from male pattern baldness which is progressive and permanent and is unlikely to be helped by therapies such as Indian Head Massage.

Patchy hair loss, or alopecia areata, is a relatively common disorder. The onset is fairly sudden and presents with a round or oval bald area; the loss of hair may be complete or so-called 'exclamation mark hairs' may be seen in the bald patches or at the edges. Occasionally the scalp is erythematous (red) in the part affected. The skin itself is not scaly, as opposed to bald areas seen in fungus infection of the scalp.

In alopecia areata there may be one or several bald patches. The most frequent course for alopecia areata to take is for the hair to regrow after a period of time (frequently two to three months). When regrowth occurs, the hair is often white but usually re-pigments in time.

Cautions, restrictions and recommendations

- Concentrate on massaging the scalp to increase the local circulation, using almond or coconut oil
- Wrap a warm towel round the head after the treatment to help aid the absorption
- Encourage the client to use the oils and massage the scalp at home twice a week, leaving the oils to absorb for about two hours before shampooing
- Advise the client of the importance of dietary requirements for healthy hair (adequate protein and essential fatty acids to promote healthy growth, and vitamin B complex and vitamin C to provide nourishment for the hair follicles; vitamin B5 helps to relieve stress).

Angina

Pain in the left side of the chest and usually radiating to the left arm. Caused by insufficient blood to the heart muscle, usually on exertion or excitement. The pain is often described as constricting or suffocating, and can last for a few seconds or moments. The patient may become pale and sweaty. This condition indicates ischaemic heart disease.

Cautions, restrictions and recommendations

- Stress predisposes an angina attack; Indian Head Massage can help to reduce stress levels by reducing the activity of the sympathetic nervous system
- As sudden exposure to extreme heat or cold can bring on an attack, keep the client warm and avoid extreme fluctuations in temperature
- It is important that clients have their necessary medications with them when they attend for treatment, in the event of an emergency.

Ankylosing spondylitis

A systemic joint disease characterised by inflammation of the intervertebral disc spaces, costo–vertebral and sacroiliac joints. Fibrosis, calcification, ossification and stiffening of joints are common and the spine becomes rigid. Typically, a client will complain of persistent or intermittent lower back pain. Kyphosis is present when the thoracic or cervical regions of the spine are affected and the weight of the head compresses the vertebrae and bends the spine forward. This condition can cause muscular atrophy, loss of balance and falls. Typically, ankylosing spondylitis affects young male adults.

Cautions, restrictions and recommendations

- Position the client according to individual comfort – extra cushioning and support may be required
- Avoid forcibly mobilising ankylosed joints, and in the case of cervical spondylitis avoid hyperextending the neck
- Gentle massage may be very beneficial and the heat generated may help to ease the pain
- Advise the client to do breathing exercises regularly in order to help mobilise the thorax.

Anxiety

This can be defined as fear of the unknown, but as an illness it can vary from a mild form to panic attacks and severe phobias that can be disabling socially, psychologically and at times physically.

It presents with a feeling of dread that something serious is likely to happen and is associated with palpitations, rapid breathing, sweaty hands, tremor (shakiness), dry mouth and general pains in the muscles. It can present with similar features of mild to moderate depression of the agitated type. The causes of anxiety can be related to personality with some genetic and behavioural predisposition, or a traumatic experience or physical illness, e.g. hyperthyroidism.

- Clients are likely to present with various symptoms and therefore a thorough assessment is required
- Indian Head Massage and relaxation exercises are likely to be a valuable source of help and support
- Clients with anxiety are more likely to become emotionally dependent on their therapist and may need to be referred to another professional for help.

Arthritis – Osteoarthritis

A joint disease characterised by the breakdown of articular cartilage, growth of bony spike, swelling of the surrounding synovial membrane and stiffness and tenderness of the joint. Is also known as degenerative arthritis.

It is common in the elderly and takes a progressive course.

This condition involves varying degrees of joint pain, stiffness, limitation of movement, joint instability and deformity.

It commonly affects the weight-bearing joints: the hips, knees, the lumbar and cervical vertebrae.

Cautions, restrictions and recommendations

- Passive and gentle friction movements around the joint may be beneficial where there is minimal pain, but excessive movement may cause joint pain and damage

- Gentle massage may help with muscle spasms, joint stiffness and muscle atrophy
- Always ask the client to demonstrate the range of movement possible in their shoulder and their neck; this will guide you as to the limitations of treatment possible.

Arthritis – Rheumatoid

Chronic inflammation of peripheral joints, resulting in pain, stiffness and potential damage to joints. It can cause severe disability. Joint swellings and rheumatoid nodules are tender.

Cautions, restrictions and recommendations

- Although Indian Head Massage cannot cure arthritis, it can help to prevent its progress through relaxation and reduction of discomfort
- In the early stages of diagnosis, clients should be encouraged to have treatment in order to maintain the range of joint movements and help prevent contractures
- In the acute stage, avoid massaging but encourage passive movement of the affected joints. In the chronic-stage treatments, massage movements can help to reduce the thickening that occurs in and around the articular cartilage
- Always ensure there is no pain and that care is taken when gently mobilising a joint
- Treatment is generally of shorter duration as clients may be taking painkillers and be unable to give adequate feedback.

Asthma

A condition in which there are attacks of shortness of breath and difficulty in breathing caused by spasm or swelling of the bronchial tubes, in turn caused by hypersensitivity to allergens such as pollens of various plants, grass, flowers, pet hair, dust mites and various proteins in foodstuffs such as shellfish, eggs and milk. Asthma may be exacerbated by exercise, anxiety, stress or smoking. It runs in families and can be associated with hayfever and eczema.

Cautions, restrictions and recommendations

- Indian Head Massage is ideally suited as a treatment for asthma sufferers as clients are seated in an upright position
- Always obtain a detailed history during the consultation stage, specifically the triggers that bring on an attack. If the client has a history of allergies then ensure that the client is not allergic to any preparations or substances you may be proposing to use
- Relaxation provided by the treatment along with deep breathing exercises can help to reduce bronchiospasm and should be encouraged
- It is advisable for the client to have their required medications handy, in the event of an attack.

Bell's palsy

A disorder of the 7th cranial nerve (facial nerve) that results in paralysis on one side of the face. The disorder usually comes on suddenly and is commonly caused by inflammation around the facial nerve as it travels from the brain to the exterior.

It may be caused by pressure on the nerve caused by tumours, injury to the nerve, infection of the meninges or inner ear, or dental surgery. Diabetes, pregnancy and hypertension are other causes.

The condition may present with a drooping of the mouth on the affected side caused by flaccid paralysis of the facial muscles and there may be difficulty in puckering the lips because of paralysis of the orbicularis oris muscle. Taste may be diminished or lost if the nerve has been affected proximal to the branch which carries taste sensations. The condition also presents with the individual having difficulty in closing the eye tightly and creasing the forehead. The buccinator muscle is also affected, which prevents the client from puffing the cheeks and is the cause of food getting caught between the teeth and cheeks. There is also excessive tearing from the affected eye. Pain may be present near the angle of the jaw and behind the ear.

Eighty to ninety per cent of individuals recover spontaneously and completely in around one to eight weeks. Corticosteroids may be used to reduce the inflammation of the nerve.

Cautions, restrictions and recommendations

- Be aware that cold and chills are known to trigger Bell's palsy
- Use light strokes in an upward direction from the middle of the face to the sides (towards the ears)
- To help increase tone on the affected side of the face, use kneading movements with the finger tips
- Light tapotement (tapping) and vibration movements may be used to help stimulate paralysed muscles
- To help maintain tone, the face massage can be performed two to three times a day
- The client may also be shown facial exercises:
  (i) To exercise the orbicularis oculi, ask the client alternately to close and open the eyes with and without mild resistance to the eyelids
  (ii) To exercise the buccinator, ask the client to puff the cheeks out and in and then try to whistle
  (iii) To exercise the orbicularis oris, the mouth should be puckered
  (iv) Saying the letters P, B, M and N helps to exercise the labials
  (v) To exercise the frontalis muscle, ask the client to raise and lower the eyebrows
- Electrotherapy (non-surgical face-lift machines or faradic) may be used to reduce the atrophy of the affected muscles.

Bronchitis

A chronic or acute inflammation of the bronchial tubes. Chronic bronchitis is common in smokers and may lead to emphysema, which is caused by damage to lung structure. Acute bronchitis can result from a recent cold or flu.

Cautions, restrictions and recommendations

- Clients with bronchitis may find Indian Head Massage more comfortable because of the fact that they are seated
- Encourage the client to breathe slowly and deeply throughout the treatment
- As sufferers of chronic bronchitis are prone to respiratory infection, therapists should avoid treating such clients if they have even the mildest form of acute chest infection.

Cerebral palsy

A condition caused by damage to the central nervous system of the baby during pregnancy, delivery or soon after birth. The damage could be caused by bleeding, lack of oxygen, or other injuries to the brain. The signs and symptoms of this condition depend on the area of the brain affected.

Speech is impaired in most individuals and there may be difficulty in swallowing. There may or may not be mental retardation.

Muscles may increase in tone to become spastic, making co-ordinated movements difficult. The muscles are hyperexcitable and even small movements, touch, stretch of muscle or emotional stress can increase the spasticity.

The posture is abnormal because of muscle spasticity and the gait is also affected. Some may have abnormal involuntary movements of the limbs that may be exaggerated on voluntarily performing a task. Weakness of muscles may also be associated with the condition, along with seizures. There may also be problems with hearing and vision.

Cautions, restrictions and recommendations

- Seek the support of the doctors, nurses, physiotherapist and the family before proceeding
- Indian Head Massage can help to reduce stress, prevent contractures, improve the circulation to the skin and muscles that are unused and provide tremendous emotional support
- Perform a shorter treatment (15–20 minutes) using mild to moderate pressure
- Since any form of stress increases the symptoms, concentrate on relaxation as this will help to reduce muscular spasms and involuntary movements
- Be aware that some clients may have reduced sensations and because of mental retardation may be unable to give adequate feedback regarding pressure and pain
- Also be aware that the spasticity in an individual may change from day to day, with changes in posture, and is related to emotional stress.

Dandruff (pityriasis capitis)

An extremely common condition which presents with visible scaling from the surface of the scalp and is associated with the presence of the yeast pityrosporum ovale. It is the precursor of seborrhoeic eczema of the scalp, in which there is a degree of inflammation in addition to the greasy scaling.

Cautions, restrictions and recommendations

- Place a clean towel over the client's shoulders when proceeding to the scalp massage, to prevent dead skin cells from the scalp falling on to their clothing
- Regular scalp massage and use of oils help to remove dead skin cells and increase the circulation
- Vitamin A is useful to improve a dry, scaly scalp.

Depression

This combines symptoms of lowered mood, loss of appetite, poor sleep, lack of concentration and interest, lack of sense of enjoyment, occasional constipation and loss of libido. On occasions there can be suicidal thinking, death wish or active suicide attempts.

Depression can be the result of chemical imbalance, usually related to serotonin and noradrenalin. The cause of depression could be endogenous where there is no cause for depression, but is thought to be linked to genetic predisposition, the result of physical illness, actual loss of a close relative, object, limb or loss of a relationship.

A depressed person looks miserable, hunchbacked and downcast, and will usually avoid eye contact.

The severity, as suggested above, can be variable but may become severe enough to become psychotic, manifested by hallucinations, delusions, paranoia or thought disorders.

Cautions, restrictions and recommendations

- A depressed client can present with physical ailments including back ache, gastro-intestinal symptoms (usually constipation) and headaches
- Physical illness can present with depression and can include, for example, long-term illness, terminal illness, Parkinson's disease and arthritis
- Therapists need to ensure that clients do not become emotionally dependent on them; they may need to be referred to another professional
- If there is any indication of suicidal thinking at any time, the client should be referred to their GP
- Indian Head Massage is thought to help increase levels of serotonin from the brain and may be effective in helping to lift depression.

Epilepsy

A neurological disorder that makes the individual susceptible to recurrent and temporary seizures. Epilepsy is a complex condition and classifications of types of epilepsy are not definitive.

GENERALISED – this may take the form of major or tonic–clonic seizures (formerly known as grand mal) in which, at the onset, the patient falls to the ground unconscious, with their muscles in a state of spasm (tonic phase). This is then replaced by convulsive movements (the clonic phase) when the tongue may be bitten and urinary incontinence may occur. Movements gradually cease and the patient may rouse in a state of confusion, complaining of a headache, or may fall asleep.

PARTIAL – this may be idiopathic or a symptom of structural damage to the brain. In one type of partial idiopathic epilepsy, often affecting children, seizures may take the form of absences (formerly known as petit mal), in which there are brief spells of unconsciousness lasting for a few seconds. The eyes stare blankly and there may be fluttering movements of the lids and momentary twitching of the fingers and mouth. This form of epilepsy seldom appears before the age of three or after adolescence. It often subsides spontaneously in adult life, but may be followed by the onset of generalised or partial epilepsy.

FOCAL – this is partial epilepsy caused by brain damage (either local or caused by a stroke). The nature of the seizure depends on the location of the damage in the brain. In a Jacksonian motor seizure, the convulsive movements may spread from the thumb to the hand, arm and face.

PSYCHOMOTOR – this type of epilepsy is caused by dysfunction of the cortex of the temporal lobe of the brain. Symptoms may include hallucinations of smell, taste, sight and hearing. Throughout an attack the patient is in a state of clouded awareness and afterwards may have no recollection of the event.

Cautions, restrictions and recommendations

- Always refer to the client's GP regarding the type and nature of epilepsy
- As epilepsy is a complex condition and Indian Head Massage involves stimulation of the brain, caution is advised
- If the client is on controlled medication, the chances of a seizure are minimal; however, caution is advised because of the complexity of this condition
- It has never been reported that holistic therapies have ever provoked the onset of epilepsy, although there is a theoretical risk to be considered in that deep relaxation or overstimulation could provoke an attack (although this has never been proven in practice).

Fibromyalgia

A chronic condition that produces musculo–sketetal pain. Predominant symptoms include widespread musculo-skeletal pain, lethargy and fatigue. Other characteristic features include a non-refreshing sleep pattern in which the patient feels exhausted and more tired than later in the day, and interrupted sleep. Other recognised symptoms include early-morning stiffness, pins and needles sensation, unexplained headaches, poor concentration, memory loss, low mood, urinary frequency, abdominal pain and irritable bowel syndrome. Anxiety and depression are also common.

Cautions, restrictions and recommendations

- Avoid deep massage on localised tender areas (which include base of skull, cervical vertebrae C5–7, midpoint of the upper border of the trapezius, above the spine of the scapula)
- Caution is advised regarding stiffness
- Relaxation is integral to reduce muscle spasm and reduce feeling of stress.

Frozen shoulder (adhesive capsulitis)

A chronic condition in which there is pain and stiffness and reduced mobility, or locking, of the shoulder joint. This may follow an injury, a stroke or myocardial infarction or may develop because of incorrect lifting or a sudden movement.

Cautions, restrictions and recommendations

If the condition is severe, refer the client to a physiotherapist. Avoid massaging the affected areas while there is acute inflammation. This condition can cause neck pain and pain at the base of the skull, which result in a headache.

Be aware that the synovial capsule of the shoulder joint will be tender and surrounding muscles and tendons will also be affected. The client will benefit from gentle stretching exercises to help mobilise the shoulder joint.

Headache (tension)

This is the most common type of headache. It involves contraction and spasm of the neck and scalp muscles. The pain is produced by the pressure of the contracted muscle on the nerves and blood vessels in the area. The resultant blood flow increases the accumulation of waste products (such as lactic acid) in the area, which perpetuate the pain.

The sufferer will usually complain of a dull, persistent ache and a feeling of tightness around the head, temple, forehead and occiput. Factors that may precipitate an attack include mental strain, noise, bright lights, alcohol consumption, menstruation and fatigue.

Cautions, restrictions and recommendations

- It is important to try to identify the precipitating cause of the headache
- Indian Head Massage is usually very successful in helping to relieve this type of headache, particularly if it is stress-induced
- Encourage the client to relax the shoulder and neck muscles with relaxation exercises before commencing the massage
- Concentrate on relaxing areas that are less tense with effleurage (smoothing/stroking) and gentle kneading and then move on to muscles which are in spasm with frictions (it is likely that these will be the neck muscles, trapezius, levator scapula and the rhomboids)
- Massage of the scalp and face can be helpful (concentrating on the temporalis muscle, the masseters and the frontalis)
- Remember that clients may be taking pain-killers and therefore may give inadequate feedback.

Kyphosis

A deformity of the spine that produces a rounded back. The condition presents with a rounded back and a flattened chest. There may be difficulty in breathing because of shortening of the pectoral muscles and the back muscles become weakened. In this condition the scapula tends to be pulled forward and the head is pushed forward.

Cautions, restrictions and recommendations

- A postural assessment is required in order to identify range of motion
- Take care with the positioning of the client and if necessary offer supporting cushions/pillows
- Concentrate on relaxing the muscles of the shoulders and neck
- Gentle stretching exercises for the back and neck may help to improve posture
- The aim of the treatment will be to relax and reduce pain in tense muscles
- Deep diaphragmatic breathing should be encouraged to help mobilise the thorax
- Avoid joint mobilisation if the condition is caused by changes in bone or connective tissue.

Migraine

Specific form of headache, usually unilateral (one side of the head), associated with nausea or vomiting and visual disturbances (usually scintillating light waves or zigzag fashion). Client may experience a visual aura before an attack actually happens. This is usually called a **classical** migraine. On occasions they cause painful, red and watery eyes – **ophthalmoplegic** migraine.

Another form of migraine can cause one-sided paralysis and weakness of the face and body; this is called **neuropathic** migraine.

Abdominal migraine can affect children, who present with recurring attacks of abdominal pain with or without nausea/vomiting.

Migraine can be treated with simple analgesics or more specialised anti-migraine medication.

Cautions, restrictions and recommendations

- Avoid treatment during acute attacks and especially if the condition has not yet been diagnosed
- Indian Head Massage is well known in helping migraine sufferers, as the relaxation and relief from stress and tension can help reduce frequency of attacks
- Remember that women are likely to have more attacks during premenstrual periods, when they are taking the contraceptive pill, during the menopause or when starting HRT
- Tension headaches can be a variant of migraine. Indian Head Massage is an ideal therapy in this event.

Myalgic encephalomyelitis (chronic fatigue syndrome)

A condition which is characterised by extreme disabling fatigue that has lasted for at least six months and is made worse by physical or mental exertion and is not resolved by bed rest. The symptom of fatigue is often accompanied by some of the following: muscle pain or weakness, poor co-ordination, joint pain, slight fever, sore throat, painful lymph nodes in the neck and armpits, depression, inability to concentrate and general malaise.

It can happen in any age group, but recently children and adolescents have been noticed to have a higher incidence.

Cautions, restrictions and recommendations

- This is a condition which can benefit from Indian Head Massage, but avoid any claim which could be misinterpreted as curative
- Relaxation can help the client to cope
- Be aware of tenderness in the muscles and joints
- Clients may require a lot of support and understanding.

Multiple sclerosis

Disease of the central nervous system in which the myelin (fatty) sheath covering the nerve fibres is destroyed and various functions become impaired, including movement and sensations. Multiple sclerosis is characterised by relapses and remissions. It can present with blindness or reduced vision and can lead to severe disability within a short period. It can also cause incontinence, loss of balance, tremor and speech problems. Depression and mania can occur.

Cautions, restrictions and recommendations

- Be aware of loss of sensation
- Be aware that massage and joint movement may trigger muscle spasm
- Relaxation therapies and exercises may be helpful in decreasing tone in rigid muscles and preventing stiffness and contractures
- Temperature extremes may make the symptoms worse
- Treatments should be slow and gentle and of short duration, as clients may tire easily.

Psoriasis (of the scalp)

A chronic skin disease which presents as erythematous (red) scaly lesions on the scalp (other common areas affected include the knees, elbows, hands, nails and the sacral area). The client with psoriasis of the scalp may complain of a severe case of dandruff. However, unlike dandruff, scalp psoriasis can be easily felt as thick plaques occurring in patches. It may cause some hair thinning which tends to recover with successful treatment of this psoriasis.

Cautions, restrictions and recommendations

See **pityriasis capitis**

Caution is advised regarding the application of oils – avoid oils which are too hot or too stimulating to the scalp (almond and coconut are good choices). Acute flare-up of psoriasis can cause painful and tender lesions of skin, and care is needed during massage. As psychological stress is a considerable cause of the exacerbation of psoriasis, Indian Head Massage can help clients to cope with their condition.

Seborrhoeic eczema (or dermatitis)

This condition presents with redness and diffuse scaling of the scalp (dandruff – see **pityriasis capitis**), which may be mild or severe. Red scaly areas may also occur on the face, especially in the eyebrows and the naso–labial folds. A similar rash may occur behind the ears.

Cautions, restrictions and recommendations

See **pityriasis capitis** *and* **psoriasis of the scalp**

Sinusitis

A condition involving inflammation of the paranasal sinuses. It is usually caused by a viral or bacterial infection or may be associated with a common cold or allergy. The congestion of the nose results in a blockage in the opening of the sinus into the nasal cavity and a build-up of pressure in the sinus.

The condition presents with nasal congestion followed by a mucous discharge from the nose. The pain is located to specific areas depending on the sinuses affected. If the frontal sinuses are affected, a major symptom is a headache over one or both eyes. If the maxillary sinuses are affected, one or both cheeks will hurt and it may feel as if there is a toothache in the upper jaw.

Cautions, restrictions and recommendations

- Be aware of the site of inflammation where there will be pain and swelling
- Pressures around the eyes and around the zygomatic bones can help to drain the sinuses and help relieve pain
- Encourage the client to drink plenty of water after the treatment to increase elimination; encourage them to consider a cleansing diet.

Stroke

A blocking of blood flow to the brain by an embolus in a cerebral blood vessel. A stroke can result in a sudden attack of weakness affecting one side of the body, caused by the interruption to the flow of blood to the brain. A stroke can vary in severity, from a passing weakness or tingling in a limb to a profound paralysis and a coma if severe. Sometimes the term is used to describe cerebral haemorrhage when an artery or congenital cyst of blood vessels in the brain bursts, resulting in damage to the brain and causing similar signs to thrombus of cerebral vessels. Haemorrhage is usually associated with severe headaches and can cause neck stiffness.

Cautions, restrictions and recommendations

- Therapists will normally deal with clients who have recovered or are recovering from a stroke and Indian Head Massage can benefit and aid recovery
- Be aware of muscle spasm and jerking movements in a paralysed limb
- Neck massage is best avoided.

Temporo–mandibular joint tension (TMJ syndrome)

A collection of symptoms and signs produced by disorders of the temporo-mandibular joint. It is characterised by bilateral or unilateral muscle tenderness and reduced motion. It presents with a dull, aching pain around the joint, often radiating to the ear, face, neck or shoulder. The condition may start off as clicking sounds in the joint. There may be protrusion of the jaw or hypermobility and pain on opening the jaw. It slowly progresses to decreased mobility of the jaw, and locking of the jaw may occur.

Causes include chewing gum, biting nails, biting off large chunks of food, habitual protrusion of the jaw, tension in the muscles of the neck and back and clenching of the jaw. It may also be caused by injury and trauma to the joint or through a whiplash injury.

Cautions, restrictions and recommendations

- Be aware that the masseter, temporalis and pterygoid muscles may be in spasm and will be tender

- The muscles of the neck, base of skull and shoulders should be massaged thoroughly to help reduce tension and spasms
- The client needs to be educated on relaxing the muscles of the jaw. Ask the client to clench the jaw firmly and concentrate on the feeling of tightness in the jaw, then relax and let the jaw fall open
- Clients may benefit from a posture assessment and breathing exercises
- Clients should be encouraged to consult their dentist and a physiotherapist for specific treatment techniques.

Tinnitis

A condition where there is the sensation of sounds in the ears or head in the absence of an external sound source. The most common cause is ordinary age-related hair cell loss in the cochlear. Other causes include wax blocking the ear canal, damage to the ear drum, diseases of the inner ear such as Ménière's disease, and abnormalities of the auditory nerve.

Cautions, restrictions and recommendations

- Indian Head Massage has been known to be effective in clearing congestion in the head and may help relieve the symptoms
- Concentrate on relaxing the neck muscle and work thoroughly above, in front of and behind the ears to increase lymph drainage
- Be aware that some clients may experience dizziness and loss of balance upon rising.

Trigeminal neuralgia

A painful condition caused by irritation of the 5th cranial nerve (the trigeminal nerve).

The condition is characterised by excruciating intermittent pain confined to one or both sides of the face, along the distribution of the trigeminal nerve. The pain may be triggered by any touch or movement such as eating, chewing, swallowing etc. Exposure to hot or cold may also trigger an attack. Some cases of facial neuralgia are caused by shingles which has healed, leaving a potentially life-long pain.

Cautions, restrictions and recommendations

- Obtain a detailed history of the signs and symptoms and refer the client to their GP before proceeding
- The client may not allow you to touch the affected side of the face
- If the client finds massage beneficial, use smoothing movements and light frictions over the skull. Then stroke gently from the middle of the face towards the temples, starting in the least sensitive area and moving gradually towards the more sensitive areas
- Do not overwork the area as it may irritate the nerve and induce pain and discomfort
- Treatment may be scheduled every other day initially.

Whiplash

A condition produced by damage to the muscles, ligaments, intervertebral discs or nerve tissues of the cervical region by sudden hyperextension and/or flexion of the neck.

The most common cause is a road traffic accident when acceleration/deceleration causes sudden stretch of the tissue around the cervical spine. It may also occur as a result of hard-impact sports. It can present with pain and limitation of neck movements with muscle tenderness which can start hours to days after the accident, and may take months to recover. This is usually affected by complicated physical, psychological and legal issues.

Cautions, restrictions and recommendations

- The condition may last for a few months or many years
- Consider compensation as a reason for delayed healing and therefore avoid making any comments about reasons, prognosis or suitability of the therapy
- Ascertain that the client is not seeking a cure; neither should the client receive any promise of doing so
- Take care when massaging the neck and avoid manipulation or moving vigorously
- Relaxation exercises can help
- Holistic therapies such as Indian Head Massage may help clients to cope with the condition
- Remember that clients with this condition would have seen many professionals and there may be legal issues you may want to avoid becoming involved with.

SELF-ASSESSMENT QUESTIONS

1   Which of the following statements is correct?

   a   alopecia is a term used to describe temporary baldness with scaly patches

   b   alopecia is a term used to describe permanent baldness with scaly patches

   c   alopecia is a term used to describe temporary baldness without scaly patches

   d   alopecia is a term used to describe permanent baldness without scaly patches.

2   Rheumatoid arthritis is

   a   a progressive disease affecting the rhomboids

   b   a chronic inflammation of peripheral joints

   c   a condition present only in elderly clients

   d   a condition also known as degenerative arthritis.

3 Bell's palsy is

   a a disorder of the 11th cranial nerve resulting in temporary paralysis on one side of the face

   b a disorder of the 7th cranial nerve resulting in temporary paralysis on one side of the face

   c a disorder of the 11th cranial nerve resulting in permanent paralysis on one side of the face

   d a disorder of the 7th cranial nerve resulting in permanent paralysis on one side of the face.

4 Which of the following statements is correct?

   a psychomotor epilepsy seizure depends on the location of the damage in the brain

   b psychomotor epilepsy was formerly known as grand mal seizure

   c psychomotor epilepsy is caused by dysfunction of the cortex of the temporal lobe of the brain

   d psychomotor epilepsy was formerly known as petit mal seizure.

5 For a client with multiple sclerosis

   a treatments should be quick and firm and of short duration, as clients may tire easily

   b treatments should be slow and gentle and of short duration, as clients may tire easily

   c treatments should be quick and firm and of longer duration, to increase clients' stamina

   d treatments should be slow and gentle and of longer duration, to increase clients' stamina.

6 If a client is suffering with sinusitis

   a avoid pressures around the eyes

   b it may feel as if there is a toothache, if the frontal sinuses are affected

   c one or both cheeks will hurt, if the maxillary sinuses are affected

   d the congestion of the nose results in a blockage in the pharynx.

Consultation for Indian Head Massage

4

A client consultation involves professional communication between a client and a therapist and is a critical skill that helps establish a positive and trusting therapeutic relationship between both parties. The time spent in establishing a professional relationship with the client will often result in client satisfaction and their continued patronage. Therapists therefore need to have effective communication skills which involve both talking and listening to clients in order to be able to record and respond positively to the information elicited.

By the end of this chapter, you will be able to:

chapter contents

- Carry out a consultation for Indian Head Massage
- Understand how contra-indications and precautions may affect the proposed treatment
- Liaise with other health care professionals
- Formulate a treatment plan for Indian Head Massage.

Client Consultation Skills

As with all holistic therapy treatments, a consultation for Indian Head Massage involves one-to-one communication. During a consultation, a therapist's contact with the client involves talking, listening and non-verbal communication, as well as the recording of written information. When carrying out a consultation, therapists need to adopt a warm, calm, open and understanding attitude towards the client, in order to facilitate a channel of positive communication.

Clients presenting for treatment may be nervous or apprehensive about the treatment and it is therefore important for a therapist to adopt a sensitive, respectful and friendly attitude to the client at all times. Although talking is an important part of a consultation, one of the most critical skills a therapist can develop is in listening. Through effective listening, a therapist can customise the treatment with the aim of meeting the client's needs and expectations. It is important for therapists to realise that clients often communicate without the spoken word and non-verbal messages may be projected without the client's awareness. Therapists therefore need to be aware of what a client may be communicating in the tone of their words, the gestures they may make, the posture they may present or by their facial expressions. With this in mind, therapists may realise that there may be a difference between what a client is expressing in words and what their body language may be indicating.

Consultation environment

In order to facilitate a positive approach to a consultation, it is important to be aware of the environment in which it is undertaken. The environment for a consultation should ideally be private in order to respect the client's privacy and dignity in disclosing personal information. Attention to aspects such as lighting, smell, temperature and comfort of a consultation area can all help to aid client relaxation and decrease apprehension.

Client education

Consultations provide an ideal opportunity for therapists to educate clients on what Indian Head Massage involves, its potential benefits along with the costs and time involved. Clients do not usually want to become passive recipients of the treatment and if they are to invest time and money in a therapy, they need to be educated so that they become partners in their healing process. Consultations also provide the client with the opportunity to ask questions about the treatment, for reassurance and clarification.

Based on the information and the education provided about the service, the client is then responsible for making a decision as to the treatment objectives. It is the therapist's responsibility to provide a treatment to suit their needs but to inform them accurately if their objectives and expectations are unrealistic. It is essential for therapists to stress to clients the importance of regular treatments to maintain long-term benefits.

Clients may also be empowered to take charge of their own healing through client education in adjustments to lifestyle, posture and the correct use of ergonomics (for example, the positioning of furniture at work).

Client confidentiality

Client confidentiality is an important factor in a therapeutic relationship between a client and a therapist. Clients should be reassured that all information recorded will remain confidential and is stored securely, and that no information will be disclosed to a third party without the client's written consent. Maintaining client confidentiality will also help to establish a trusting professional relationship between a client and a therapist.

Written documentation

Written documentation is essential in a consultation as it provides a systematic and continued record of the client's progress. Consultation documents should always be used as a guide to facilitate communication, and questions may need to be phrased in a certain way to maximise communication and receive qualitative information. For instance, upon asking a client about their stress levels, they may merely reply 'High'. In order to gain more information, a therapist may pose the question 'In which part of the body do you feel stress most often?' or 'What factors are involved in your stress levels being high at the moment?'.

It is important for therapists to realise that information received from the client is largely subjective in that it is from their viewpoint, and this information may differ from what is evaluated by the therapist.

Important information to be discussed during the consultation are any factors which may affect the client's physical and emotional health, such as medical history, diet, lifestyle, occupation, sleep patterns, exercise and relaxation, which may all contribute to an overall picture of the client from a holistic point of view. Besides talking, listening and recording information on a client's records, client consultation involves other assessment skills such as:

- **visual assessment** – this commences from the first point of contact with the client. Observations as to the client's mood, rate and depth of breathing, posture and gait may all help to contribute to assessment of the state of the client's physical and emotional health
- **manual assessment of the tissues** – the most effective form of communication a therapist can facilitate is in touch, and throughout the Indian Head Massage treatment the therapist can assess the tissues for tension, restrictions, temperature changes etc.

Contra-indications and Cautions

Despite Indian Head Massage being an extremely safe and effective treatment, it is important for therapists to be aware of:

a conditions that are totally contra-indicated and for which treatment cannot be provided

b conditions that require referral to the client's GP or another professional before treatment may be given

c conditions that present as localised contra-indications, therefore treatment should be avoided in the affected area

d additional cautions which may affect the proposed treatment plan.

Knowledge of contra-indications and precautions enables a therapist to work safely and effectively.

A) Conditions that are totally contra-indicated to Indian Head Massage

These include:

- **fever/high temperature** – this is a contra-indication because of the risk of spreading infection as a result of the increased circulation. During fever, the body temperature rises as a result of infection
- **acute infectious diseases** (for example, colds, flu, measles, mumps, tuberculosis, chicken pox) – acute infectious diseases are contra-indicated because they are highly contagious
- **skin or scalp infections** – these should be avoided because of the risk of cross-infection. Some of the most common skin diseases that may be encountered on the head and neck include: herpes simplex (cold sores), impetigo, ringworm, scabies, conjunctivitis, folliculitis, pediculosis capitis (head lice) and tinea capitis (ringworm of the scalp)
See pages 23–30 for more detail on these and other skin and scalp disorders.

- **recent haemorrhage** – haemorrhaging is excessive bleeding which may be either internal or external. Indian Head Massage should be avoided due to the possibility of increasing the risk of blood spillage from blood vessels
- **intoxication** – it is inadvisable to carry out treatment while a client is under the influence of alcohol, as the increase of blood flow to the head could make them feel dizzy and nauseous
- **migraine** – it is inadvisable to carry out treatment if a client indicates the onset of an attack of migraine, because they may become nauseous or dizzy or experience visual disturbances with severe headache and possible vomiting. In reality, clients experiencing an acute attack of migraine will usually be incapacitated by its effects and would be unable to receive treatment, let alone desire a treatment, at the time of the attack. *However, Indian Head Massage may help as a preventive treatment, particularly if the migraine is stress-induced*
- **recent head or neck injury** – in the case of a recent blow to the head with concussion, or an acute neck injury caused by a recent accident, such as whiplash, it would be inadvisable to treat because of the risk of exacerbating the condition and increasing the inflammation and pain. However, if there is an old injury, massage may help to reduce scar tissue, decrease pain and increase mobility. Always obtain medical advice to ensure the client's condition is suitable for treatment.

B) Conditions that may be contra-indicated to Indian Head Massage, but require medical advice before deciding whether treatment is advisable

- **severe circulatory disorders/heart conditions** – medical advice should always be sought before massaging a client with a severe heart condition or circulatory problem, as the increased circulation from the massage may overburden the heart and can increase the risk of a thrombus or embolus. *If medical advice indicates that massage is advisable, it is recommended that a lighter massage is given, of a shorter duration initially*
- **thrombosis/embolism** – always seek medical advice before massaging a client with a history of thrombosis or embolism, as there is a risk that the blood clot could become detached and be carried to another part of the body where it could obstruct the flow of blood to a vital organ. *If medical advice indicates that massage is advisable, it is recommended that a lighter massage is given, of a shorter duration initially*
- **high blood pressure** – clients with high blood pressure should have medical referral prior to massage, even in they are on prescribed medication, because of their susceptibility to forming clots. Clients on anti-hypertensive medication may be prone to postural hypotension and may feel light-headed and dizzy after treatment. Therapists are advised to monitor a client's reaction carefully and to advise clients to get up slowly from the chair following treatment. *If medical advice indicates that massage is advisable, techniques applied are generally soothing and relaxing*
- **low blood pressure** – care should be taken with a client suffering from low blood pressure when sitting or standing up after massage, because they may experience dizziness and could fall
- **dysfunction of the nervous system** – clients with any dysfunction of the nervous system should be referred to their GP before treatment is given. A light, relaxing massage may be indicated

in the case of a client with cerebral palsy, multiple sclerosis or Parkinson's disease as massage may help to reduce spasms and involuntary movements and reduce rigidity and stiffness. *Always seek medical advice before offering treatment*

- **epilepsy** – always refer to the client's GP regarding the type and nature of epilepsy from which the client suffers. Caution is advised because of the complexity of this condition and the risk that deep relaxation or overstimulation could provoke a convulsion (although this has never been proven in practice). *As some types of epilepsy may be triggered by smells, care should be taken with choice of oils or medium*

- **diabetes** – this is a condition which requires medical advice, as some clients with diabetes may be prone to arteriosclerosis, high blood pressure and oedema. Pressure should be monitored and administered carefully, because of the possibility of loss in sensory nerve function resulting in the client being unable to give accurate feedback regarding pressure. *If the client is receiving insulin by injection, care should be taken to avoid massage on recent injection sites. Clients should have their necessary medications with them when they attend for treatment, in case of an emergency*

- **cancer** – medical advice should always be sought before massaging a client with a cancerous condition. There is a risk of certain types of cancer spreading through the lymphatic system; massage is also thought to aid in the metastasis of the cancer. It is unlikely that gentle massage can cause cancer to spread through the stimulation of lymph flow, but it is important always to obtain advice from the consultant/medical team concerning the type of cancer and the extent of the disease. Once medical advice has been obtained, massage may help in relaxing the body and supporting the immune system. It may also be used in palliative care (therapy that eases or reduces pain or other symptoms). *If massaging a cancer patient, always avoid massage over areas of the body receiving radiation therapy, close to tumour sites and areas of skin cancer. It is usual to offer short, light massage, which is beneficial in relaxing the client and supporting the immune system*

- **recent operations** – depending on the nature of the operation and the area/s affected, it may be necessary to seek medical advice before proceeding with treatment. If a client has recently undergone surgery to the head or neck, Indian Head Massage should be avoided as it may interfere with the healing process. Medical advice is often necessary to establish when the area has completely recovered

- **osteoporosis** – because bones can break easily and vertebrae can collapse with this condition, it is advisable to seek medical advice before giving treatment. *If medical advice indicates that treatment is advisable, care needs to be taken in ensuring comfortable client positioning, avoiding excessive joint movement and applying a lighter pressure.*

C) Conditions that present as localised contra-indications

- **skin disorders** – care should be taken as the condition may be worsened. Some skin conditions such as eczema, dermatitis and psoriasis should be treated as a localised contra–indication, as affected areas may be hypersensitive and the condition may be exacerbated by massage

- **recent scar tissue** – massage should be applied only once the tissue is fully healed and can withstand pressure. Gentle frictions may be applied over healed scar tissue in order to help break down adhesions

- **severe bruising, open cuts or abrasions** – these should be treated as localised contra–indications, and if presented in the treatment areas they should be avoided
- **undiagnosed lumps, bumps and swellings** – the client should be referred to their GP for a diagnosis. Massage may increase the susceptibility to damage in the area by virtue of pressure and motion.

D) Additional cautions

- **allergies** – care should be taken to ensure that any oils or products used do not contain items to which the client may be allergic. Patch tests should be carried out to avoid adverse reactions
- **asthma** – care should be taken to position the client comfortably during treatment, and to avoid using any massage mediums or substances to which a client may be allergic
- **medication** – certain medications may inhibit or distort the client's response to give feedback regarding pressure, discomfort and pain. Always check with the client's GP if you are unsure as to type of medication and its effects
- **pregnancy** – although pregnancy is not strictly a contra-indication, unless there are serious complications, special care should be taken for a pregnant client to ensure that they are comfortable during the treatment. Therapists should be aware that some women may experience side-effects as a result of the pregnancy, such as dizziness and high blood pressure. Pressure and duration of treatment may need to be adjusted according to the individual circumstances.

Liaising with other Health Care Professionals

As the benefits of Indian Head Massage become more widely known and validated, there are more opportunities opening up for therapists to work alongside other health care professionals. Therapists therefore need to be aware of professional and medical etiquette when liaising with other professionals.

Referral to a health care professional

If a contra-indication is established with a client at the time of consultation, treatment cannot usually proceed without reference to the client's GP. In this case, it is helpful to have a pre-prepared referral form on headed notepaper that may be taken by the client to their doctor, or may be posted with a stamped addressed envelope.

Example of Referral Form

Therapist's Name

Clinic Address

Date

Doctor's Address

Surgery

Dear Doctor _____

I am writing with regard to one of your patients_____ of

_____

who has requested Indian Head Massage treatment *(please see attached information on Indian Head Massage)*.

Your patient has informed me that he/she suffers from *(high blood pressure etc)*

Please can you advise me in your medical opinion if there is any reason why this patient should not receive an Indian Head Massage?

Thank you for your assistance in this matter.

Therapist's name and signature

Doctor's advice note

The proposed treatment of Indian Head Massage you suggest would be suitable/unsuitable for this patient.

Doctor's name and signature

When referring to a client's GP, it is important to note that a doctor's insurance will not cover them for giving permission or consent to holistic therapy treatments. It is therefore essential that therapists make it clear that they are seeking advice about the client's medical condition, in order to decide whether Indian Head Massage treatment is suitable, and that their proposed treatment is in accordance with medical advice.

In order to raise awareness of Indian Head Massage amongst doctors and other health care professionals, it is important for a therapist to include literature on Indian Head Massage, concerning its methodology, benefits and effects.

Handling referral data from other health care professionals

If a client has been referred to a therapist by another health care professional, it is professional etiquette to reply with a status report on the client's progress. Report writing is an essential part of networking with other professionals, as it helps to raise awareness of the benefits of the treatment and its value to a client's physical and emotional wellbeing.

A status report should include the following information:

* a general introduction to the client and how he or she was referred
* a summary of the client's main presenting problems
* an evaluation of the therapist's findings
* the treatment used and explanation of the techniques involved
* the client's progress
* recommendations for future/continued treatment.

The most important factor in the consultation, besides whether the client is medically suitable for treatment, is their expectations of and objectives for the treatment.

Setting professional boundaries

In order to have a healthy and professional relationship with clients, there should be a balance between care and compassion for the client, and keeping a distance from any personal involvement.

The setting of boundaries can provide the foundation upon which a therapist can build a professional relationship with a client. A therapeutic relationship should always involve distance between a therapist and a client, in order to make it safe for both parties. There is always a risk of transference in a client–therapist relationship, in which a client begins to personalise the professional relationship and thus steps over the professional boundary. There is also the risk of counter-transference, when a therapist has difficulty in maintaining a professional distance from the client's problems and begins to step into a friend/counsellor role. If either of these situations occurs, it is important for a therapist to realise how potentially damaging this can be for a client and themselves, and how it detracts from their healing process.

When to refer a client to another member of a health care team

While Indian Head Massage can be very beneficial in relaxing a client and relieving minor stress-related conditions, it is important to realise that all treatments have their limitations.

If a client presents a condition that is beyond the scope of their treatment, such as a serious medical physical or psychological condition, it is essential that a therapist is able to recognise this and to refer the client to another professional who can best help them. In this instance, it is useful for therapists to have resources available for clients to access, such as information on:

- other complementary therapies
- counsellors or psychotherapists
- professional therapy organisations whom members of the public can contact for details of qualified members
- advice centres
- self-help groups.

Displaying information affords the client the choice of picking their own suitable way of moving forward with their own situation.

Holistic therapy treatments such as Indian Head Massage always tend to work best when there is a combined treatment strategy; this may involve a client receiving regular treatments, making lifestyle adjustments and attending for treatment with another health care professional.

On the following page is an example of a consultation form that may be used for Indian Head Massage.

Indian Head Massage Consultation Form

Client note

The following information is required for your safety and to benefit your health. While Indian Head Massage is a very safe treatment, there are certain conditions which may require special attention.

This information will be treated in the strictest of confidence and it may be necessary for you to consult your GP before treatment can be given.

Date of initial consultation: _____   Client ref. no. _____

Personal details

Name: _____   Title: Mr/Mrs/Miss/Ms/Other: _____

Address: _____

_____

Telephone number: _____(evening)   _____ (daytime)

Date of birth: _____   Occupation: _____

Medical details

Do you have/have you ever suffered from: (please give dates and details)

			Dates and Details
High temperature or fever?	Y	N	_____
Acute infectious disease?	Y	N	_____
Skin infections?	Y	N	_____
Recent haemorrhage?	Y	N	_____
Are you currently under the influence of alcohol or drugs?	Y	N	_____
Recent head or neck injury?	Y	N	_____
Recent surgery?	Y	N	_____
Severe circulatory disorder?	Y	N	_____
Heart condition?	Y	N	_____
Thrombosis/embolism?	Y	N	_____
High or low blood pressure?	Y	N	_____
Dysfunction of the nervous system?	Y	N	_____
Epilepsy?	Y	N	_____
Diabetes?	Y	N	_____
Any potentially fatal/terminal condition?	Y	N	_____
Recent scar tissue?	Y	N	_____
Severe bruising, open cuts or abrasions?	Y	N	_____
Undiagnosed lumps, bumps or swellings?	Y	N	_____
Allergies?	Y	N	_____

Migraine or headaches?   Y   N   _____

Scalp infection?   Y   N   _____

Female clients

Is it possible that you may be pregnant?   Y ( )   N ( )

Are there any other conditions you have which may affect the proposed treatment?

Y ( )   N ( )

Details _____

_____

Are you currently taking any medication?   Y ( )   N ( )

Details (including dosages) _____

_____

Is GP referral required?:   Y ( )   N ( )

Clearance form sent: Y ( )   N ( )   Date:_____

Clearance form received: Y ( )   N ( )   Date:_____

Name of doctor: _____   Surgery: _____

Address: _____

Telephone number: _____

Lifestyle

Is your general health/immunity:	Good ( )	Average ( )	Poor ( )
Are your stress levels:	High ( )	Medium ( )	Low ( )
Are your energy levels:	High ( )	Medium ( )	Low ( )
Do you find time for relaxation/hobbies:	Y ( )	N ( )	

Details: _____

Client declaration

I declare that the information I have given is correct and, as far as I am aware, I can undertake treatments without any adverse effects. I have been fully informed about contra-indications and am therefore willing to proceed with treatment. I understand that Indian Head Massage is not a substitute for medical treatment.

Client signature: _____   Date: _____

Formulating a Treatment Plan for Indian Head Massage

Once the verbal and non-verbal information has been elicited from the client, the therapist is then in a position to suggest a treatment plan, or strategy, and obtain the client's agreement before proceeding.

A treatment plan for Indian Head Massage will include the following information:

- the date of the treatment
- feedback from any previous treatment, if applicable
- any updated information on the client's condition since the original consultation
- the treatment objectives
- client expectations
- any special considerations, such as specific areas to be worked on, special needs or requirements
- an outline of the proposed treatment, to include areas for treatment, length and cost of treatment
- suggested treatment frequency (this may also be reviewed at the end of the treatment)
- type of oils used (if applicable) and reasons for choice
- the client's agreement.

key note

An important consideration in a client's treatment plan may be the time of day the treatment is undertaken. A client may require the treatment in the morning to awaken the nerves gently and to prepare the body for the day's activities, or may require the appointment later in the day to help remove the stresses of the day and promote sleep.

Treatments should be reviewed at regular intervals in order to monitor progress and elicit client satisfaction. By discussing a treatment plan regularly with a client, their individual needs can be taken into consideration and changes can be made, if necessary.

Example of a Treatment Plan for Indian Head Massage

Client's name: Chris Parkin   **Date of treatment:** 19th September

Proposed treatment: Indian Head Massage treatment of all areas, concentrating on neck and shoulders because of tension. Client has recently had a head cold and has been experiencing sinus congestion.

Time of treatment: early evening app't required – 6.30pm

Treatment timing: 30 minutes

Cost: £22.00

Client expectations

- To feel calm and more relaxed
- To improve sleep pattern
- To reduce muscular tension in the neck and shoulders
- To help relieve sinus congestion.

Treatment objectives

- General stress relief and relaxation
- Concentrate on reduction of muscular tension in the neck and shoulder regions
- Concentrate on relieving sinus congestion with pressure points to the face.

Special client considerations

As the client's posture is poor because of occupational stress, consideration needs to be given to client comfort and client awareness (advice to be given on basic stretches to improve posture). Client's stress levels are high presently, so emphasis will be on relaxation and good breathing throughout.

Oils to be used

Coconut oil to be used for dry scalp condition.

Recommended treatment frequency

Because of the client's high stress levels at present, it is recommended that treatment is commenced at weekly intervals for a month and then reviewed.

SELF-ASSESSMENT QUESTIONS

1 Which of the following is the most critical skill needed for a therapist to carry out an effective consultation for Indian Head Massage?

   a talking

   b being friendly

   c showing empathy

   d listening.

2 What action should be taken if, during a consultation, a client informs you that they have very high blood pressure?

   a offer a lighter treatment which is soothing and relaxing

   b proceed with a normal treatment but keep checking that the client doesn't feel dizzy

   c ask the client to seek advice from their GP to see if treatment is advisable

   d do not offer a treatment unless the client is taking medication.

3 Which of the following conditions would indicate that Indian Head Massage treatment could not be offered?

   a recent scar tissue

   b low blood pressure

   c acute infectious disease

   d open cut or abrasion.

4 Which of the following conditions would not require referral to a GP for advice before offering treatment?

   a thrombosis/embolism

   b dysfunction of the nervous system

   c recent head or neck injury

   d open cut or abrasion.

5 Why is it important to avoid using the words 'permission' or 'consent' on a doctor's referral note?

   a it is unethical

   b the correct medical terminology must be used for insurance purposes

   c it is not professional etiquette

   d a doctor's insurance will not cover them for giving permission or consent to holistic therapy treatments.

Indian Head Massage Case Studies

As part of the development process for therapists studying to become professional practitioners of Indian Head Massage, it is necessary to carry out a number of case studies to explore the practical efficacy of the techniques and, most importantly, to gain valuable practical experience of the skills learned.

Carrying out several treatments on case studies encourages repetitive practice and can help to increase confidence levels through client feedback.

This chapter is devoted to providing general guidelines on how to approach case studies, along with three examples.

By the end of this chapter, you will:

chapter contents

- Know how to present an Indian Head Massage case study as part of an assessment for a professional qualification.

Indications for Treatment

There are many conditions which a client may present that may benefit from Indian Head Massage.

Common conditions with which Indian Head Massage has been known to help include:

- tension headaches
- eyestrain
- muscular tension
- emotional stress
- anxiety and depression
- insomnia and disturbed sleep patterns
- sinusitis
- poor hair condition.

What is a Case Study?

As part of the professional training for Indian Head Massage, you will be required to complete and present a number of case studies for assessment.

A case study is a record of a series of treatments carried out on a client, which has been evaluated for effectiveness.

Outlined below are some general guidelines on how to present case studies.

When considering whom to choose for your case studies, it is necessary to choose as wide a range of clients as possible in order to meet the requirements of a professional award and to prepare you for commercial practice.

The essential components of a case study are as follows:

Client profile

This is a general introduction to the client and will include background information such as age range, occupation, lifestyle issues, sleep patterns, hobbies and interests, along with their main presenting problems/any factors that may affect them in their daily life.

Consultation form

Before any treatment commences, the client needs to be assessed in order that their individual considerations may be taken into account (health problems or special needs).

A full consultation must be carried out and recorded, which will include personal, medical and lifestyle details, along with a declaration and the client's signature.

See the example of an Indian Head Massage Consultation Form on pages 96–97.

Observations

These may include initial and ongoing observations from information elicited from the original consultation and subsequent treatments. Therapists need to be perceptive of non-verbal signs the client may exhibit, such as their posture, facial expressions and breathing rate. These are all factors which will not be evident from the recording paperwork. The noting of these factors will assist the reader or assessor to build a fuller picture of your case study, and will reflect the development of your perceptive skills.

Treatment plan

Once the initial consultation has taken place, a course of treatment may then be recommended.

A treatment plan will typically include the following information:

- client's name
- date and time of treatment

- outline of proposed treatment and areas to concentrate on
- treatment timing
- cost
- client expectations
- treatment objectives
- special client considerations
- oils to be used
- recommended treatment frequency.

Record of treatments

It is important that a record is kept of all treatments carried out. This will typically include:

- an assessment of the client's physical condition (noting any areas of tension, physiological responses) as well as psychological responses and body language (e.g. client nervous or apprehensive)
- visual assessment of the client (noting posture, non-verbal signs)
- any known reactions, their effects and any advice given
- after care advice given
- home care advice, along with any oils or products suggested for home use
- outcome and general evaluation of the treatment
- recommendations for future treatment and the suggested frequency.

Evaluation

Evaluation is an essential part of a case study, as it is only through feedback and evaluation that a therapist can gauge the effectiveness of the treatments given, and ultimately measure their own professional development.

Factors to consider in evaluating the treatment with the client are:

- Was the course of treatments effective. If so, in what ways?
- What benefits, if any, were derived from the treatments?
- Were there any particular parts of the treatment the client liked or disliked?
- Were there any contra-actions?
- Is the client keen to continue with regular treatments?

Written testimonial

Once the course of treatments has been completed, it is necessary, for the purposes of assessment and authenticity, to ask your case study clients to complete a written testimonial, which is a handwritten letter to confirm that they have received a course of treatment on the dates concerned; it should outline any benefits they have noticed as a result.

Self-evaluation

It is also important for therapists to carry out their own self-evaluation, in order to assess their own development. By critiquing performance, therapists can perfect their skills and commit to continual improvement.

Examples of Case Studies

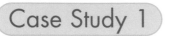
Case Study 1

Client profile
Name: Jan
Age: 42 years
Occupation: mature student and homemaker

Jan is a mature student with two girls of 17 and 14 years of age. She is currently training to be a counsellor and is currently on work placement at a local doctor's surgery.

Her life is therefore very busy, looking after her two daughters, completing her studies and looking after their home. Despite her busy schedule, Jan does find some time to relax; she swims, goes for walks and loves reading.

Physically, Jan is fit and healthy, with no medical conditions. However, she does sometimes feel stressed out because of the pressure of her studies and running a home. She finds her neck muscles are often tight; in particular, the right trapezius muscle often aches, causing her a degree of discomfort.

Jan's energy and stress levels are average.

Treatment objectives
Jan had never experienced Indian Head Massage before. The effects and benefits of the treatment were therefore explained to her.

After consultation, it was agreed with Jan that the treatment objectives were to:

* help relieve muscular tension in the shoulders and neck
* aid general relaxation and relief of tension
* help uplift Jan psychologically and aid stress relief.

Treatment plan
It was agreed with Jan that a course of three treatments would be given over a period of two weeks; the first two were given in a week, and the third in the following week.

Coconut oil was to be used on the scalp as Jan's hair and scalp have a tendency to dryness.

Account of treatments

Treatment 1

On commencement of the first treatment, Jan indicated that she was very tired mentally, as she had just returned from her work placement.

The treatment uncovered a lot of tension in the neck and shoulder area. The neck and shoulders were very stiff. A lot of deep breathing was suggested throughout the treatment, to help ease tension.

By the time we reached the scalp massage Jan was almost asleep.

After the treatment, Jan reported that at the start she was aware of all her thoughts and her mind was not still. However, at the end of the treatment she felt calm and extremely relaxed but at the same time energised.

Jan was advised to take plenty of water following treatment, to rest, to have a light meal and to avoid alcohol or caffeine consumption. She was also encouraged to leave the oil on for a few hours following treatment before shampooing.

Jan did not have any adverse reactions after the treatment and reported that she felt quite energetic the next day.

Treatment 2

The second treatment was given three days after the first. Jan had been at college all day and was tired, but less tension was noticeable. She relaxed from the beginning and fell asleep. At the conclusion of the treatment, she felt relaxed, calm and contented.

Jan did not report any adverse reactions after her second treatment and reported that she felt relaxed but energetic the next day.

Treatment 3

The third treatment was given a week later. During this treatment, Jan commented on the overall improvement she was experiencing and how the muscular tension had decreased to the point where it no longer caused her discomfort. She reported that she was also feeling more relaxed and energetic.

Outcomes and recommendations

The course of three treatments has proved very beneficial to Jan. During and after each treatment, the improvements have been visibly noticeable. Jan has also commented enthusiastically on how much better she has felt.

Further treatments were recommended to maintain Jan's progress and condition and it was suggested that treatments were continued once fortnightly as a preventive measure against tension build-up.

Client testimonial

'The experience of the head was quite different from anything I had experienced before. I was aware of my tension during the first treatment and found the shoulder and upper arm movements quite strange. However, the pressure was just right and by the second and third treatments I knew what to expect and was much more relaxed. In the second and third treatments I actually fell asleep – something I never realised I could do sitting upright in a chair!

I think I slept better and definitely felt more invigorated in the days afterwards, and less tense.

I really enjoyed and appreciated the experience and shall definitely be continuing with regular treatments.'

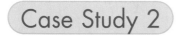

Case Study 2

Client profile
Name: Pam
Age: 79 years
Occupation: retired librarian

Pam is a widow with two daughters and four grandchildren whom she looks after on a regular basis. Although Pamela is retired, she enjoys quite an active social life, playing tennis, swimming and enjoying gardening.

Generally, Pam is in good health and has no major illnesses, but sometimes suffers from sinusitis, headaches and disturbed sleep. She takes HRT and cholesterol tablets for which she has regular reviews with her GP.

During the consultation, Pam revealed that she had had manipulation on her left shoulder under anaesthetic two years ago. However, Pam's current condition did not prove to be contra-indicated to treatment, although caution was observed when treating the shoulder and upper arm area. She did not present with any other conditions or considerations for treatment.

Generally, Pam has low levels of stress and medium energy levels, but recently has been feeling low energy levels. When explaining the benefits, Pam mentioned her dry scalp and thinning hair.

Treatment objectives
After consultation, it was agreed that the treatment objectives were to:

- aid general relaxation
- reduce congestion in the sinus area
- improve scalp and hair condition
- relieve muscular tension
- improve energy levels.

Treatment plan

It was agreed with Pam to give a course of three treatments over a four-week period. The first and second treatments would be weekly and the third after a fortnight.

Account of treatments

Treatment 1

Pam has never had any form of massage treatment before and was quite apprehensive. As a result, she was unable to relax fully during her first treatment. She enjoyed the scalp massage and felt that the pressure points over the sinus area on the face had helped to ease congestion. Pam commented that she felt relaxed at the conclusion of the treatment.

Pam reported that she felt calm and she experienced no adverse reactions the next day.

Treatment 2

During this treatment, the muscles in Pam's neck and upper back felt very tight. She explained that this was because of gardening she had carried out during the day. Deep breathing was advised, to help ease tension during the treatment. Pam was visibly more relaxed during this session and commented that her neck and upper back felt better.

Pam reported that she experienced a headache for a couple of days after the second treatment; this she felt was caused by congestion and the sinuses.

Treatment 3

The third treatment was given two weeks later. During the treatment, Pam commented on how the pressure points over the sinus area had helped and how the use of oil had helped with the dryness of the scalp and hair. Pam relaxed really well during this treatment and almost fell asleep.

After-care advice was given after each treatment: to drink plenty of water, to rest, to have a light meal and to avoid consumption of alcohol and stimulants. Pam was also shown some simple massage techniques with oil to use at home for the long-term care of the hair and scalp condition.

Outcomes and recommendations

The course of treatments has been successful for Pam. She felt relaxed after each treatment and indicated how the treatments have helped with her sinusitis, sleep pattern and her hair and scalp condition. Pam also commented on how her energy levels have improved since treatments commenced.

Pam has requested that she continue with regular treatments for relaxation and body maintenance. Suggested frequency is once a fortnight.

Client testimonial

'The course of Indian Head Massage I have received has been a beneficial and new experience for me. Having never received a massage, I was unsure of what to expect and felt quite nervous to start with.

Everything was so well explained, and the pressure was perfect for me. Although I felt relaxed after the first treatment, I was able to relax more fully on the second and third, knowing what to expect. I would very much like to continue with regular treatment, as this seems an ideal way to relax. It has certainly helped to improve my sinusitis and headaches, and after each treatment I found I slept more soundly and woke feeling more refreshed.'

Case Study 3

Client profile
Name: Kelly
Age: 18 years
Occupation: student

Kelly is completing her A levels in maths and the sciences. She is fit and in good health, but suffers from hay fever for which she takes antihistamines.

Kelly has never experienced Indian Head Massage before; however, because of exam stress she was keen to try the treatment for stress relief and relaxation.

Treatment objectives
After consultation, it was agreed with Kelly that the treatment objectives were to:

- help relieve muscular tension
- help relieve mental fatigue
- promote psychological uplift
- aid relaxation and stress relief.

Treatment plan
It was agreed with Kelly that because of her high stress levels at exam time, two treatments would be given in the first week and the third treatment given a week later.

Account of treatment

Treatment 1

During the first treatment, Kelly was unable to relax to start with. However, she began to relax with the neck massage and actually feel asleep during the scalp massage. A lot of tension was found in the neck and shoulder muscles. A little more time was devoted to treating the shoulder area and Kelly was advised to take plenty of deep breaths throughout the treatment, to help ease tension.

Kelly was quite surprised by how relaxed the treatment had made her feel and commented that she could not believe she fell asleep sitting up. She felt calm, relaxed and energetic at the end of the first treatment.

She was advised to drink lots of water, to rest, to eat a light meal following treatment and to avoid consumption of alcohol and stimulants.

Treatment 2

The second treatment was carried out after four days. Kelly reported that after the first treatment she felt relaxed and a bit tired the next day, but became more energetic as the day went on.

At the commencement of the second treatment, Kelly's neck and shoulders felt much looser. During the treatment she relaxed and fell asleep, but during the face massage she was awake and alert. After treatment, she was keen to go to an aerobics class, but was advised against it to rest, in order that the energy could be utilised in the body for the healing process. After-care advice was given as for after the first treatment.

Treatment 3

The third treatment was given a week later. Kelly reported that she had had a slight headache the day after the second treatment, but also felt more calm and relaxed. She commented that she had also felt dehydrated and felt better after drinking more water.

During the third treatment, Kelly fell asleep soon after the treatment started but remained awake and energetic during the face massage.

After-care advice was specified as in previous treatments.

The day following the third treatment, Kelly reported that she felt quite tired and lethargic in the morning. She also felt dehydrated but felt better after drinking more water. She commented that, as the day progressed, she felt much more energetic.

Outcomes and recommendations

The series of treatments given has been successful for Kelly. She felt she was able to relax, unwind and relieve her mental fatigue caused by the pressure of the exams.

After each treatment, Kelly felt tired, lethargic and dehydrated because of toxins being released. However, after drinking more water Kelly felt much better – energetic, calm and relaxed.

Kelly is keen to continue treatments for relaxation; suggested frequency would ideally be once a fortnight.

Client testimonial

'I thoroughly enjoyed my head massage sessions. I had never experienced a head massage before and found some of the sensations quite strange for the first time, yet at the same time they were very relaxing. While my back, shoulders and arms were being massaged I felt very lethargic and fell asleep every time these areas of my body were massaged. However, I found that when my neck, scalp and face were massaged I felt very energised and revitalised. The massage always left me feeling energetic and lively, yet calm and relaxed inside. During each massage I was aware that my body was relaxing, my heart rate slowed slightly and I fell asleep very easily as I became used to the movements. I also noticed that during the massage I was unaware of time passing, as I was so relaxed.

The days following the massages I sometimes felt quite tired and lethargic. I was also slightly dehydrated, but soon felt better when I increased my intake of water.

I feel the head massage sessions have enabled me to relax and cope with my increased stress levels at this time and therefore I feel I have really benefited from the treatments. I would also like to continue with the treatments regularly, to maintain the benefits.'

Indian Head Massage Techniques

In India, massage has long been adopted as a daily practice in order to help maintain a healthy mind and body throughout the course of life. In the modern day of high stress levels in the Western world, massage is a must for relaxing both mind and body, and recharging depleted energy levels. Indian Head Massage is uniquely different from other types of therapeutic massage practised in the West in that it is applied through the clothes, to a client in a seated position, thereby supplanting the need for special or sophisticated equipment.

By the end of this chapter, you will be able to:

chapter contents

- Understand the massage movements used in Indian Head Massage, along with their effects
- Prepare a treatment area for Indian Head Massage
- Understand the properties and benefits of oils and herbs used in Indian Head Massage
- Carry out a step-by-step Indian Head Massage treatment to the upper back and shoulders, upper arms, neck, scalp and face
- Provide after-care advice.

Massage Movements used in Indian Head Massage

The massage techniques used in Indian Head Massage are simple but extremely effective. They consist of a combination of traditional Indian techniques and Westernised techniques.

Effleurage

Effleurage is one of the principal techniques used in Indian Head Massage. It is a stroking, or *smoothing* movement that signals the beginning and end of a massage. Effleurage is also used as a linking movement to facilitate the flow from one technique to another. Effleurage is applied with the whole hand, fingers or the forearms. Pressure can be superficial or deep, depending on the effects to be achieved. Effleurage can be applied slowly and gently to produce a calming and soothing effect or applied more briskly to stimulate the circulation and energise and revitalise the person being massaged. In Indian Head Massage a combination of slow, gentle stroking and brisker energetic effleurage is used.

Effects of effleurage

Effleurage:

- dilates the capillaries and increases the circulation
- relaxes the client by soothing sensory nerve endings in the skin
- prepares the area for deeper strokes
- aids in moving waste out of congested areas
- soothes tired, achy muscles
- warms the tissues, making them more extensible.

Petrissage

Petrissage movements are deeper movements using the whole hand, thumbs or fingers. There are many types of petrissage used in Indian Head Massage (picking up, squeezing and releasing, rolling etc.). Petrissage movements involve the skin and muscular tissue being moved from their position and squeezed with a firm pressure away from the underlying structure and then released.

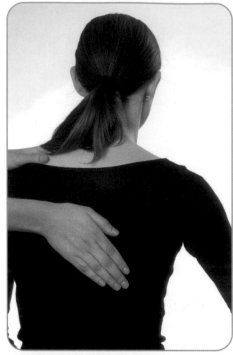

Effleurage

Effects of petrissage

Petrissage:

- increases the removal of waste products from the tissue and encourages fresh oxygen and nutrients to be delivered to the tissues
- stretches muscle tissue and fascia
- reduces adhesions and muscular spasms
- relaxes muscle tissue and reduces accumulated stress and tension from the muscles.

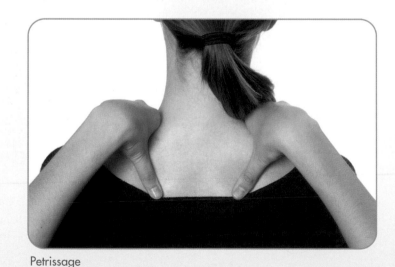

Petrissage

Tapotement

These techniques are performed with the fingers and are similar to percussion movements in Swedish massage. They involve a series of light, brisk, springy movements applied with both hands in rapid succession.

The main tapotement movements used in Indian Head Massage are as follows:

- **hacking**: this technique involves flicking the hands rhythmically up and down in quick succession, using the ulnar borders of the hands
- **champi**: this technique is also known as 'double hacking'. It is performed by holding the hands in a prayer position, and allowing them to relax so that the heels of the hands and the pads of the fingers and thumbs are gently touching. A series of light, rapid striking movements is then performed across areas such as the shoulders
- **tabla playing (tapping)**: 'tabla' refers to a drum used in the classical and popular music of Northern India. It is a light technique that uses the fingertips to tap on the head.

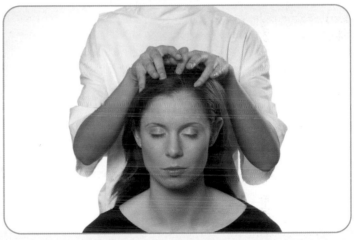

Champi

Tabla playing

Effects of tapotement

Tapotement:

- stimulates the nerve endings
- increases the circulation and local blood flow
- increases muscle tone through stimulation of muscle fibres
- wakens and refreshes the body.

When applied lightly, these strokes are soothing and bring about relaxation and a release of tension; when applied more deeply they have a stimulating effect on the nerves and are refreshing.

Frictions

A strong feature of the Indian Head Massage is friction movements which are performed with the whole of the hand, the heel of the hand, the fingers or the thumbs. They are deeper, more penetrating movements that cause the skin to rub against the underlying structures. Frictions are excellent for breaking down tension nodules that have accumulated because of stress and tension. Frictions are particularly useful in Indian Head Massage for working around the scapulae and on either side of the spine.

Effects of frictions

Frictions:

- dilate the capillaries and increase the circulation
- generate heat locally in the area massaged
- loosen stiffness and tension by relaxing muscles
- break down and help free adhered tissue in restricted areas.

Vibrations

These are fine shaking, trembling or oscillating movements that are applied with one or both hands, using either the whole palmar surface of the hand or the fingertips. A fine trembling movement may be achieved by moving the fingers up and down or side to side while maintaining contact with the skin. Vibrations may be performed either in a static form or where the hands or fingertips travel over a point while still vibrating. Vibration movements may be fine, deep or vigorous, depending on the effect required.

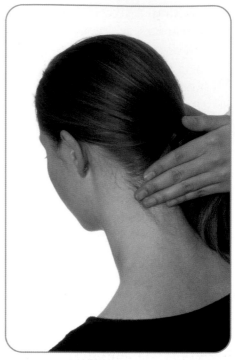

Frictions

Effects of vibrations

Vibrations:

- help relieve tension and aid relaxation, creating a sedative effect
- stimulate and clear nerve pathways, creating a refreshing effect
- stimulate muscle spindles, thereby creating minute muscle contractions
- help relieve pain.

Pressure points

Pressure points are vital energy points similar to acupressure used in Chinese medicine. In Ayurveda it is said that the 'life force' is located in the head.

Balancing the energy within these vital points will promote health at all levels within the body. The stimulation of pressure points in the head is said to stimulate the hypothalamus, pituitary and other areas of the brain to promote healing to be relayed to various parts of the body.

Effects of pressure points

Pressure points are applied with the fingers and the thumbs, and they:

- clear congestion in the nerve pathways
- relieve pressure and pain from tense muscles
- relieve sinus congestion

- encourage lymph drainage
- increase circulation locally to the area
- restore the energy balance to the body.

Marma points

Marma points are an integral part of Ayurveda and are the subtle pressure points, similar to points used in acupressure, that stimulate the life force or *pranic* flow. The marmas are anatomical places on the body, mostly composed of flesh and bones.

There are a total of 107 marmas in the body:

- 37 in the head and neck
- 12 in the front of the body
- 22 in the upper limbs
- 14 in the back of the body
- 22 in the lower limbs.

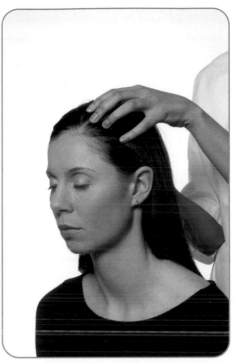

Pressure points

Marma points are naturally sensitive points that are measured by finger widths, known as *anguli*. The finger width is the finger of the person being treated and not the therapist's own finger. The location of marmas is given in this way because each person is made differently and has a different size and proportion. The location of marmas may vary from one to eight finger widths, and often relates to regions of the body and not a point.

In Indian Head Massage the marmas may be used to:

- treat the pranas
- treat a specific organ or system of the body
- treat a specific dosha imbalance.

Marma points relating to the head and neck

Marma point	Size	Quantity	Location	Composition	Treatment use
Adhipati	4 finger widths	1	top of head	joints in skull	control of mind, nerves and prana vayu
Simanta	linear placement	5	on joints of skull bones	joints in skull	control of nerves and prana vayu
Shringatakani	½ finger width	4	soft palate	blood	control of nerves and prana vayu
Sthapani	½ finger width	1	between eyebrows	blood vessels	control of mind, nerves, endocrine glands and prana vayu
Utkshepa	½ finger width	2	above *Shankha*	ligament	control of large intestine and apana vayu
Shankha	2 finger widths	2	temple between ear and *Apanga*	bone	control of large intestine and apana vayu
Avarta	½ finger width	2	above eyebrows on the sides	joint	controls vision, alochoka pitta and prana vayu
Apanga	½ finger width	2	corners of the eyes	blood vessels	controls vision, alochoka pitta and prana vayu
Phana	½ finger width	2	both sides of the nostrils	blood vessels	controls the sinus and prana vayu
Vidhura	½ finger width	2	below both ears	tendon	controls hearing, balance, and prana vayu

Marma point	Size	Quantity	Location	Composition	Treatment use
Krikatika	½ finger width	2	junction of head and neck	joint	release neck and shoulder tension and udana vayu
Sira Matrika	4 finger widths	8	4 arteries on each side of the neck	arteries	circulation of the blood to the head and heart, vyana vayu
Nila	4 finger widths	2	on each side of the larynx	blood vessel	circulation, hoarse voice, udana vayu
Manya	4 finger widths	2	back of *Nila*	blood vessel	control of blood, circulation and vyana vayu

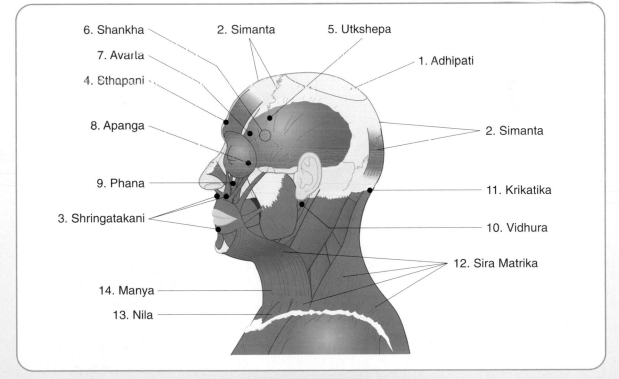

Marma points

Treatment methods of marma points

Marma points may be treated with pressure, circular massage, heat and with oils. Pressure is used on the marmas in the same way as any other form of pressure therapy. The marma is first found and located by the practitioner, finding a hard, tender or sensitive point. Pressure is then increasingly applied with conscious breathing, in the knowledge that prana is going out from the fingers and into the client. When enough pressure has been applied, small counter-clockwise massage movements may be used to break up the tension from the point.

In general, clockwise movements stimulate or energise a marma point and a counter-clockwise movement dispels and liberates blocked or stagnant prana.

The key to using pressure therapy on a marma point is to go slowly and deeply and to work within the comfort zone of the client. It is essential to avoid pushing forcibly through a marma, as this can go against the internal harmony and interfere with the healing process.

Health and safety note

Although the treatment of marma points is part of traditional Ayurvedic massage, it is essential that practitioners receive additional professional training and study in order to promote safe and effective use of them, as any incorrect application or injury to these subtle energy points can cause danger to life.

Compression

This is a form of petrissage in which the muscles are gently pressed against a surface such as the scalp, top of the shoulders or the upper arms, with the palms of both hands, and then slowly released.

In general, the effects of compression are:

- increased blood flow locally to the area being treated
- through gentle compression of the blood vessels and nerves, tension may be relieved in the muscles and pain is alleviated.

Hair tugging

This is a technique used in the scalp massage where the roots of the hair are lifted and pulled upwards, in between the fingers of both hands. The effect of hair tugging is to stimulate hair growth through the nerve stimulation to the hair root.

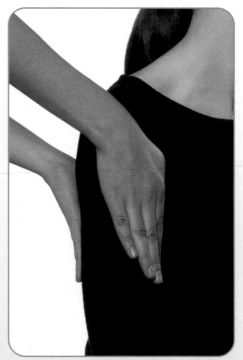

Compression

Equipment and Materials for Indian Head Massage

The beauty of Indian Head Massage lies in its simplicity. It can be performed in an ordinary chair, without the need to purchase expensive equipment.

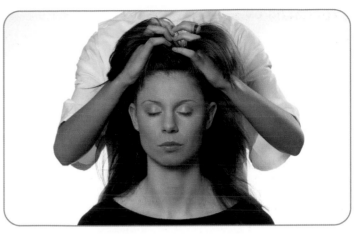

Hair tugging

- The type of chair best suited to Indian Head Massage treatments is one with a relatively low back and without an arm rest.
- An important factor for the therapist is the height of the chair; it is therefore preferable for the therapist to work with a chair with an adjustable height and back rest to ensure correct body mechanics.

It is also important for a therapist practising Indian Head Massage to have a variety of oils for optional use on the scalp, and a hand cleanser. The types of hand cleanser most suited to a visiting therapist are dry anti-bacterial cleansers which are easy and practical to use.

Oils used in Indian Head Massage

The use of oil is optional when massaging the scalp. Oil that is applied to the head is absorbed into the roots of the hair which are connected with nerve fibres leading to the brain.

Applying oil to the head helps to strengthen the hair and remove dryness and, by relaxing the muscles and nerves of the head, fatigue is eliminated, leaving the recipient feeling refreshed and revitalised.

Massaging the head increases the fresh supply of oxygen and glucose to the brain and improves the circulation of spinal fluid around the brain and the spinal cord.

There are several oils which may be used for Indian Head Massage.

Traditionally, oils such as sesame, coconut, olive, mustard and almond have been used by Indian women as part of their grooming ritual, to keep their hair in good condition.

key note

When the body is subjected to stress and illness, the skin and hair are often affected, resulting in dryness and sometimes loss of hair. With tension, the scalp becomes tight, restricting the flow of nutrients to the hair that promote healthy hair growth. Using oils on a regular basis can help to encourage healthy shiny hair, slow down hair loss and soften and moisturise the hair.

- **Almond oil** – being high in nutrients such as unsaturated fatty acids, protein, vitamins A, B, D and E, this oil makes an excellent hair conditioner, helping to soften, moisturise and protect the hair. This oil has warming effects on the body and is therefore useful for stimulating hair growth, as well as helping to reduce muscular pain and tightness.
  Caution: avoid this oil if your client has an allergy to nuts.

- **Coconut oil** – this is a popular oil for Indian Head Massage and is widely used in southern parts of India, especially in the spring. It is a light oil which is very moisturising and softening on the skin and the hair. It also helps to relieve inflammation and can be useful for dry, brittle hair and hair that has become lifeless because of chemical and physical stress.
  Caution: take care with hypersensitive skin.

- **Mustard oil** – this oil is often found in Indian grocery stores and is one of the most popular oils used in north-west India. It is especially used during the winter months because of the hot, warming sensation it creates. The smell is strong and pungent and its effects are very warming by increasing body heat. It is a popular oil among wrestlers and bodybuilders in India. Mustard oil is well known for its ability to break down congestion and swellings from tense muscles and to relieve pain. For dryness of the scalp, using mustard oil with a small amount of turmeric powder can prove very effective.
  Caution: this oil may irritate the skin because of its stimulating nature.

- **Olive oil** – this oil is very popular in the Western world. It is of viscous consistency with a strong smell and is therefore often mixed with another lighter oil such as almond. The virgin or extra virgin variety of this oil contains high levels of unsaturated fatty acids and can therefore be useful in helping to moisturise dry skin and hair. It has excellent moisturising properties and is soothing and penetrative. It has stimulating properties which help to increase heat in the body and is therefore helpful to reduce swellings and alleviate muscular tightness and pain.

- **Sesame oil** – this is one of the most popular oils used in the western part of India. It is used as a base oil for all oils used in head massage and is very popular in Ayurveda. Sesame seeds are high in minerals such as iron, calcium and phosphorus which help to strengthen, nourish and protect the hair. Sesame seed oil is excellent for dry skin and hair. It can also help to improve skin texture, reduce swellings and alleviate muscular pain. It is particularly popular in India during the summer as it does provide some protection from the rays of the sun.

Note: the oils used in Indian Head Massage are seasonal, with mustard and olive being a popular choice in the winter because of their warming effects and sesame and coconut being more popular in the summer months.

In addition to the oils mentioned above, there are other oils which are traditionally used in India for the treatment of hair. These oils are blended with Eastern herbs and spices not readily available in the West. These may be imported and sold in traditional Indian supermarkets and health stores.

- **Amla oil** – in combination with henna, this is an excellent hair tonic. It promotes the growth of healthy and lustrous hair and has a cooling and nourishing effect.

- **Brahmi oil** – this is a unique combination of carefully selected exotic herbs blended with pure coconut oil. Brahmi oil is used medicinally in India as a tonic for the nervous system for those suffering from anxiety and emotional exhaustion. Brahmi oil helps the growth of long, lustrous hair and provides relief from dandruff and joint pain. It is also said to help improve the memory and dispel mental fatigue.
- **Bhringraj oil** – this is a popular oil for daily head and scalp massage in India. As well as helping to promote hair growth, it is said to nourish brain cells, help encourage better sleep and relieve stress and tension.
- **Neem oil** – this oil is native to India and has antiseptic, astringent and anti-bacterial properties. Early Sanskrit medical writings refer to the attributes of neem. It is particularly effective for relieving itching and irritation, on the scalp and the skin.
- **Pumpkin seed oil** – this oil is extremely nourishing for dry and stressed hair, as pumpkin seeds are rich in vitamins A, E, C and K, unsaturated fatty acids and proteins.
- **Shikakai oil** – this is an excellent hair rejuvenator and has astringent and antiseptic properties. Is said to help with eczema and dry scalp.

The use of essential oils in Indian Head Massage

Traditionally, essential oils such as sandalwood, jasmine and rosemary have long been used in India as part of Ayurvedic preparations. While the properties of essential oils can be extremely beneficial on the hair and the scalp, it is recommended that essential oils are not individually blended by a therapist practising Indian Head Massage unless they are qualified and insured for the practice of selecting and blending essential oils. Many essential oil suppliers have pre-blended preparations for sale which may be used in Indian Head Massage. However, caution is advised on safe proportions because when carrying out Indian Head Massage you are close to the brain and the olfactory response, and therefore the effects of essential oils may be enhanced.

Significant Points on the head for oil application in Indian Head Massage

There are three important points on the head, according to the Ayurvedic tradition:

- The **first point** can be found by measuring eight finger widths above the eyebrows. This is where it is recommended that oil is poured onto the scalp initially and then distributed symmetrically down both sides of the head with the fingers.
- The **second point** is at the crown of the head on the mid-line: an important therapeutic point, this is where blood vessels, nerves and lymphatics meet. Oil is traditionally poured onto the crown and then evenly distributed down the sides of the scalp.
- The **third point** is at the base of the skull and is the point where the neck meets the skull. Oil is traditionally poured onto this point, with the person's head inclined forwards, and is then mixed in either side and towards the ears.

Chakra Balancing and Indian Head Massage

Chakras

Everything that happens to us on an emotional level has an energetic impact on the subtle body, which in turn has an impact on the physical body. Chakras are non-physical energy centres located about an inch away from the physical body. The energy field of each chakra extends beyond the visible body of matter, into the subtle body or aura.

It is important to remember that chakras do not have a physical form and any illustration of the chakras is merely a visual aid to the imagination and not a literal, physical reality.

Chakras are a way of describing the flow of subtle energy and are often said to be related to an endocrine gland, which the chakra is thought to influence. With stress, the chakras can lose their ability to synchronise with each other and become unbalanced. If negative energy becomes stored in a chakra, it can accumulate and the function of the chakra becomes impaired. Ultimately this can lead to energy blocks where the chakra virtually ceases to function and creates an imbalance as other chakras attempt to compensate for the blocked centre, creating additional strain for the energy system.

The effects of an accumulation of negative energy in the chakras can manifest themselves as an emotional or physical condition. Often we are only aware of a change in the physical body as our attention is drawn to it in the form of pain or disease; this may not always be linked to being a symptom of a cause within the subtle body.

Chakras are the focal points for the energies of the subtle bodies and are the key to restoring balancing. By placing hands along the axis of the chakras, energy can be aligned and harmony restored. By working with the subtle energy of the chakras, energy may be strengthened, decreased or balanced as needed by the body at the time of the treatment.

The base or root chakra (Muladhara)

Location – at the base of the spine.

Relevance – it is the foundation chakra and is linked with nature and planet Earth. It is concerned with all issues of a physical nature – the body, the senses, sensuality, a person's sex, survival, aggression and self-defence. At a physical level, it is linked to the endocrine system through the adrenal glands. Its energies also affect the lower parts of the pelvis, the hips, legs and feet.

Imbalance – if this chakra is unbalanced it can make a person feel as if they are ungrounded and unfocused. They may feel weak, lack confidence and feel unable to achieve their goals.

Colour association – the colour to visualise in balancing the base chakra is red.

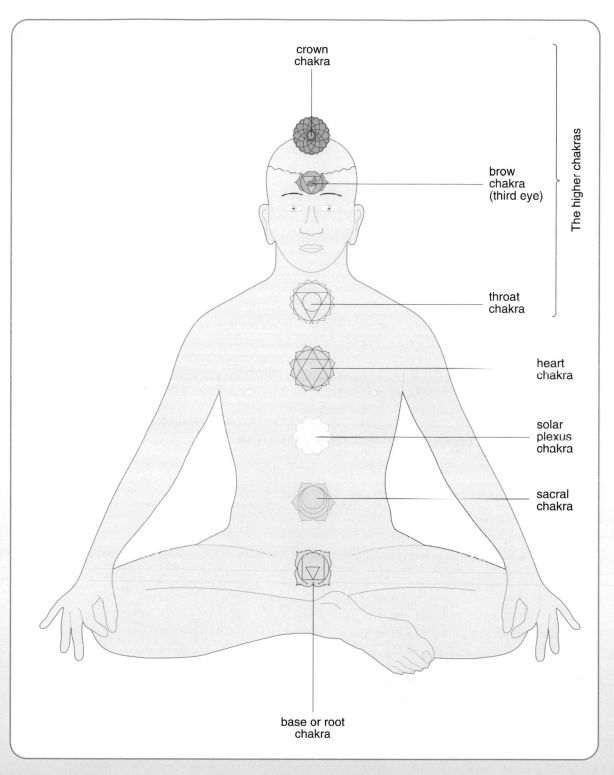

crown
chakra

brow
chakra
(third eye)

The higher chakras

throat
chakra

heart
chakra

solar
plexus
chakra

sacral
chakra

base or root
chakra

Seven major chakras

The sacral chakra (Swadhistana)

Location – at the level of the sacrum, between the navel and the base chakra.

Relevance – concerned with all issues of creativity and sexuality. At the physical level, it is linked to the testes in the male and the ovaries in the female. Its energies also affect the urino–genital organs, the uterus, the kidneys, the lower digestive organs and the lower back.

Imbalance – a person with an imbalance in this chakra may bury their emotions and be overly sensitive. An imbalance may also lead to sexual difficulties and energy blocks with creativity.

Colour association – the colour to visualise in balancing the sacral chakra is orange.

The solar plexus chakra (Manipura)

Location – at approximately waist level.

Relevance – this chakra relates to our emotions, self-esteem and self-worth. Feelings such as fear, anxiety, insecurity, jealousy and anger are generated here. At a physical level, it is linked to the Islets of Langerhans in the pancreas. Its energies also affect the solar and splenic nerve plexuses, the digestive system, the pancreas, liver, gall bladder, diaphragm and middle back.

Imbalance – people who are under a degree of stress will show imbalance in this chakra; shock and stress have a greater impact on this chakra than on others. It is in the solar plexus chakra that negative energies relating to thoughts and feelings are processed. People with an imbalance in this chakra may feel depressed, insecure, lacking in confidence and may worry what others think.

Colour association – the colour to visualise in balancing the solar plexus chakra is yellow.

The heart chakra (Anahata)

Location – in the centre of the chest.

Relevance – this chakra is concerned with love and the heart. It deals with all issues concerned with love and affection. At a physical level it is linked to the thymus gland. Its energies also affect the cardiac and pulmonary nerve plexuses, the heart, lungs, bronchial tubes, chest, upper back and arms. It is also the point of connection between the upper and lower chakras.

Imbalance – if the energy does not flow freely between the solar plexus and the heart, or between the heart and the throat, this can lead to some form of imbalance because of the energy withdrawal into the body. A person with an imbalance in this chakra may feel sorry for themselves, be afraid of letting go, feel unworthy of love or feel terrified of rejection.

Colour association – the colour to visualise in balancing the heart chakra is green.

The throat chakra (Vishuddha)

Location – at the base of the neck.

Relevance – this chakra is concerned with communication and expression; it also deals with the issue of truth and true expression of the soul. At a physical level, it is linked to the thyroid and parathyroid glands. Its energies also affect the pharyngeal nerve plexus, the organs of the throat, the neck, nose, mouth, teeth and ears.

Imbalance – if this chakra is out of balance it may result in the inability to express our emotions; if unexpressed feeling is bottled up it can lead to frustration and tension. A person with an imbalance in this chakra may feel unable to relax.

Colour association – the colour to visualise in balancing the throat chakra is blue.

The brow chakra (Ajna)

Location – in the middle of the forehead, over the 'third eye' area.

Relevance – commonly known as the 'third eye', the brow chakra is the storehouse of memories and imagination and is associated with intellect, understanding and intuition. At a physical level, it is linked to the hypothalamus and pituitary gland. Its energies also affect the nerves of the head, brain, eyes and face.

Imbalance – if this chakra is not functioning correctly it can lead to headaches and nightmares. A person with an imbalance in this chakra may be oversensitive to others' feelings, be afraid of success, be non-assertive and undisciplined.

Colour association – the colour to visualise in balancing the brow chakra is indigo.

The crown chakra (Sahasrara)

Location – on top of the head.

Relevance – this chakra is the centre of our spirituality and is concerned with thinking and decision-making. At a physical level, it is linked to the pineal gland. Its energies also affect the brain and the rest of the body.

Imbalance – an imbalance in this chakra may be reflected in those who are unwilling or afraid to open up to their own spiritual potential. An imbalance may also show as being unable to make decisions.

Colour association – the colour to visualise in balancing the crown chakra is violet.

key note

An important part of Indian Head Massage treatment is the Eastern tradition of balancing the higher chakras (the throat chakra, the brow chakra or third eye and the crown chakra).

With stress and tension, the chakras lose their ability to synchronise with one another and become unbalanced.

By placing the hands along the axis of the higher chakras, energy can be realigned and a sense of balance and harmony can be restored.

Preparation for an Indian Head Massage Treatment

Client preparation

- Check client is suitable for treatment, by carrying out a consultation.
- Formulate the client's individual treatment plan.
- Seat client comfortably in a chair, ensuring that their legs are uncrossed and feet are placed on the ground.
- Drape a towel over the back of the chair and have a clean towel ready for placing over the shoulders for the scalp massage.
- Ask the client to remove any obtrusive jewellery such as necklaces, earrings and noserings, and to remove glasses.
- Ask the client to brush their hair to remove any residue of hairspray and mousse, and to remove face make-up.
- If the client's hair is long, it should be tied up with a suitable clip.

Therapist preparation

- Present a smart and professional appearance.
- Tie hair back off the face.
- Remove all obtrusive jewellery and wrist watch.
- Ensure chair height is at a suitable height for you and your client.
- Prepare oil for the scalp massage, if required (approximately 2–5ml, depending on the length of the hair and the condition of the scalp). The oil application is often preferable when applied to the scalp warm. If this is desired, place the oil container in a bowl of warm water before treatment.

Hygiene precautions

- Cleanse hands before and after treatment.
- Check client for any infectious conditions.
- Avoid carrying out treatment if you have any infection which may be transmitted.

- Cover any open cuts or abrasions with a waterproof plaster.
- Pour oil into a separate container for individual client use and dispose of residual oil.

Correct body mechanics

Body mechanics involve the correct use of posture in order to apply Indian Head Massage techniques with the maximum efficiency and with the minimal trauma to the therapist. Therapists often find it more difficult initially adjusting from massaging a client on a couch to massaging a client while they are seated in a chair. It is therefore essential that correct adjustments are made to body mechanics in order to increase the effectiveness of the massage, help prevent repetitive strain injuries, decrease fatigue and increase comfort for the therapist.

Guidelines for correct body mechanics include:

- checking chair height – a chair at the correct height will enable a therapist to use body weight effectively to develop pressure
- wearing low-heeled shoes with good support
- keeping the back straight by tilting the pelvis forwards
- using body weight effectively, by lunging in order to create pressure needed
- keeping the shoulders and upper back relaxed (avoiding raising shoulders to ears)
- keeping feet firmly placed on the ground
- bending knees slightly and keeping knees soft, taking care to avoid locking them straight
- keeping wrists as straight as possible
- avoiding joint hyperextension
- keeping the body in correct alignment by maintaining head erect over neck and shoulders
- keeping head forward posture to a minimum and avoiding spending too much time looking down
- taking breaks in between clients to stretch the neck, shake out the arms and relax
- varying the massage techniques used and varying hand and foot placements
- having regular treatments in order to keep body working at an optimum level.

Adaptations to an Indian Head Massage Treatment

Indian Head Massage, like any other massage techniques, should always be adapted and varied to suit the differences in the physical characteristics of the client, such as their body size, muscle tone, age and hair characteristics.

Therapists are likely to encounter many different clients who may require a degree of adaptation because of their physical and health-related situations.

key note

The best approach to massage is to see every client's situation as a different challenge and view their individual needs as part of the treatment plan.

When adapting a massage it is not the massage movements themselves that change; the difference is in the way in which the therapist modifies or adjusts the pressure, speed, duration and frequency of the massage.

A pregnant client

It is advisable to avoid carrying out Indian Head Massage in the first trimester, until the pregnancy is established. The first trimester can be an unsettling time and some clients may experience nausea and sickness.

Once past the first trimester, and provided the pregnancy has no complications, Indian Head Massage can often be a popular choice because pregnant clients can sit comfortably in a chair for treatment, and no special positioning is required.

Care should be taken when massaging a pregnant client because some clients may experience a feeling of dizziness. Care should also be taken, and if necessary GP referral sought, for those clients who experience high blood pressure during their pregnancy.

A disabled client

The first consideration for the therapist is to establish the nature of the disability, and if necessary research the condition beforehand, in order to be prepared. It is important for a therapist to enquire tactfully about the limitations of the condition and not to assume anything; just because a client is disabled does not mean that they are paralysed.

If a client is in a wheelchair, then because of the portability of Indian Head Massage they may be treated quite easily while sitting in the wheelchair. In this case it is advisable for the therapist to sit or kneel when carrying out the consultation in order that they may talk to the client at eye level.

It is essential to take care with disabled clients not to appear patronising, as many disabled clients may be very fit and able and should not be discriminated against because of their disability.

An elderly client

There are several considerations to be borne in mind with an elderly client.

* Take care to ensure the client is warm enough throughout the treatment.
* Many elderly people experience a sudden drop in blood pressure, so care needs to be taken to help the client up to avoid falls and losing balance.

- Avoid deep massage because of decreased reaction time, possible insensitivity to pain and thinning of skin and blood vessels.
- There may be loss of hearing and vision.
- There will be a decrease in muscle tone and bones will not be as strong and flexible; joints may be worn.
- Skin may appear pale, wrinkled, become thinner, looser and more frail.
- The circulation may not be as efficient, especially if the client is inactive.

It is best to make the treatment sessions shorter, as the client may tire easily, and to take care when applying pressure and avoid extreme joint mobilisation because of the loss of bone integrity.

A large-framed client

Clients with a large frame may find Indian Head Massage more comfortable because of the positioning and the fact that no undressing is required.

Pressure should be applied carefully to areas with dense areas of adipose tissue, in order to avoid tissue damage and client discomfort. It may be tempting for the massage therapist to consider that areas of fatty tissue are insensitive and to apply too firm a pressure. Adipose tissue is in fact highly vascular, making it very susceptible to bruising and damage. General pointers are to consider pressure and to monitor client feedback and use body mechanics correctly.

The therapist may also need to adjust the chair height, depending on the size of the client.

A small-framed client

Care needs to be taken with a thin client to avoid deep massage or pressure over bony areas which may cause discomfort. Stimulating techniques such as hacking should be avoided over unprotected areas, and pressure applied carefully monitored in line with client feedback.

It is important for the therapist to avoid assuming that because the client is thin they require a light massage; pressure applied should be carefully monitored in line with client feedback.

In general terms, the male body presents more muscle bulk than the female body and therefore an adaptation of technique is often required. Male clients will generally require a firmer pressure and the therapist should take care to apply the correct body mechanics and posture in order to be able to carry out the techniques effectively and to the client's satisfaction.

Adaptations for clients without hair

Clients without hair will require a slightly different approach when massaging the scalp. Any techniques involving manipulation or tugging of the hair will obviously be omitted. However, it is still important to work over the scalp, as regardless of whether the client has hair, the scalp muscles are still liable to develop tension because of their attachments.

Indian Head Massage Techniques

An Indian Head Massage treatment typically consists of massage to the upper back and shoulders, upper arms, neck, scalp and face. Treatment is traditionally applied through the clothes, with the use of oil being optional on the scalp. Illustrated below is an example of a step-by-step routine of Indian Head Massage treatment.

Because they have been taught through families for generations and have been Westernised, it should be noted that techniques may vary in their content and application.

The shoulders

The shoulders are the place where most people hold a considerable amount of tension. When the body is in a state of tension the shoulders are lifted towards the ears and often remain this way, causing the muscles to go into spasm. This restricts the blood flow to the head, neck and shoulders and causes the neck and shoulders to become stiff and inflexible. Sitting with hunched shoulders can reduce chest capacity and thus impair breathing.

> *key note*
>
> Indian Head Massage can help to counterbalance the effects of stress, as by relaxing the shoulders they will drop and allow the energy to flow more freely to the area, encouraging deeper and easier breathing and improved joint flexibility.

Upper back and shoulder massage

1. STARTING POSITION with hands over the top of the client's shoulders

Therapist's stance

Standing behind the client, in a relaxed posture.

Technique

- Commence by holding your hands lightly on your client's shoulders.
- Ask your client to take three deep breaths, with the emphasis on breathing in and out slowly and deeply.

> *key note*
>
> This helps the client and therapist relax and prepare themselves for treatment.

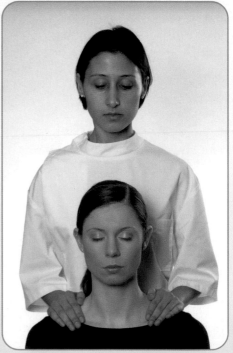

Starting position

2. HOLDING POSITION over the top of the head

Therapist's stance

Standing behind the client, in a relaxed posture.

Technique

- Hold your hands lightly on either side of the head for about a minute, waiting for a feeling of relaxation and calm.
- You are now ready to commence the massage.

> ### key note
>
> This helps to create a feeling of stillness and calm before commencing the massage.

3. EFFLEURAGE/SMOOTHING across the shoulders and upper back

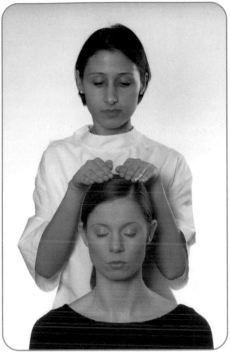

Holding position

Therapist's stance

Standing behind the client, in a walk standing position. Therapist uses walk standing posture to lunge forward and increase the pressure and effectiveness of the techniques.

Technique

- Use one hand to support one side of the upper back.
- Use the palmar surface of the other hand to stroke up either side of the spine, across the top of the shoulder and around the lateral border of the scapula to return to the starting position.
- The stroke upwards should be deeper than the stroke downwards.
- Repeat three times one side and then repeat the other side, gradually increasing in pressure with each stroke.

> ### key note
>
> This technique is the first communication across the shoulders and enables the therapist to establish contact and feel for any areas of tension.

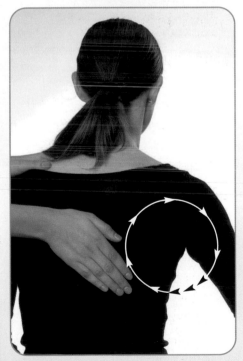

Effleurage/smoothing

4. PETRISSAGE/THUMB SWEEPING across the shoulders

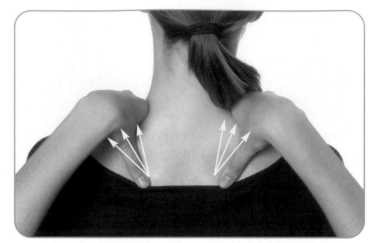

Petrissage

Therapist's stance

Standing behind the client, in a walk standing position. Therapist uses walk standing posture to lunge forward and increase the pressure and effectiveness of the techniques.

Technique

- With fingers resting on the top of the client's shoulders, reach down the upper back with your thumbs and place them as far as they can go either side of the spine, across the lower border of the trapezius muscle.
- Now draw the thumbs up and across the trapezius muscle, fanning out towards the little finger.
- Repeat three times, gradually increasing in pressure.
- Now draw the thumbs up towards the middle finger and repeat three times.
- Then draw the thumbs up towards the index finger and repeat three times.

key note

This is a deeper technique that helps to unlock tension and free fibrous adhesions from the trapezius muscle.

5. FRICTIONS WITH THE HEEL OF THE HAND, rubbing around the scapulae

Therapist's stance

Standing to the side so that you are facing your client's shoulder from the side.

Technique

- Support one side of the back with one hand.
- Use the *heel* of your other hand to rub lightly and briskly (in a side-to-side motion) across the top of the scapulae, in between the scapulae and below the scapulae, in the characteristic 'C' shape.
- Repeat three times on each side.

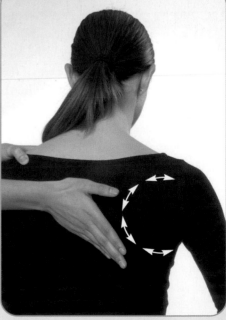

Frictions

> **key note**
>
> This technique creates a considerable amount of heat in the tissues and helps to break down fibrous adhesions and restrictions around the scapulae.

6. FRICTIONS WITH THE FINGER, rubbing around the scapulae

Therapist's stance

Standing to the side so that you are facing the client's shoulder from the side.

Technique

- Support one side of the back with one hand.
- Join the fingers of the other hand and place fingertips so that they face away from the spine.
- Rub vigorously backwards and forwards across the top of the scapulae, in between and below the scapulae, in the characteristic 'C' shape.
- Repeat three times on each side.

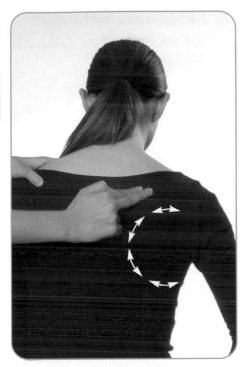

Frictions with the finger

> **key note**
>
> This technique is similar to the previous technique, in helping to free restrictions and tension from around the scapulae.

7. SMOOTHING EFFLEURAGE (repeated as in 3)

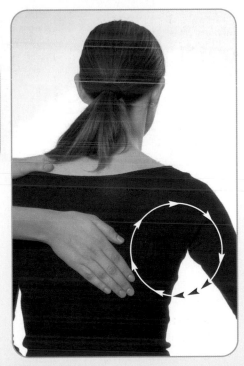

Effleurage/smoothing

8. PRESSURES with the knuckles either side of the spine

Therapist's stance

Standing behind the client, in a walk standing position.

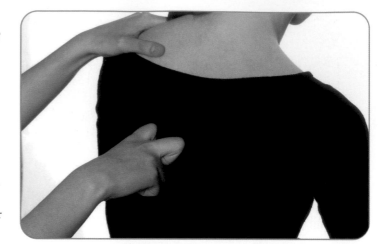

Pressures with the knuckles

Technique

- Place the middle knuckles of the forefinger *and* middle finger on either side of the spine, at the top of the shoulders.
- Ask the client to take a deep breath in and *as they breathe out*, apply pressure inwards and then slowly release back towards you.
- Continue working down either side of the spine, approximately an inch at a time, until you reach the mid-spine.
- Lightly sweep back up to the top of the shoulders, and repeat two times.

key note

This technique stimulates the nerve endings either side of the spine, releasing blockages in the nerves and easing tension.

9. THUMB PUSHES over the shoulders

Therapist's stance

Standing behind the client, in a walk standing position.

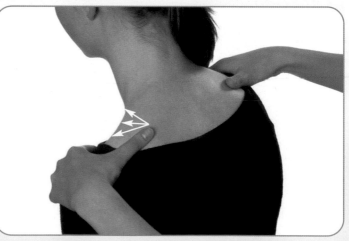

Thumb pushes

Technique

- Place the palms of the hands around the cap of the shoulder (deltoid muscle), with thumbs resting above shoulder blades.
- Starting from the outer edge of the shoulder, use the pads of the thumbs to push in one long sweep from the trapezius muscle (back of the shoulders) over to the pectoralis major muscle (front of the chest).

- Slowly release and then move further in towards the neck, and repeat.
- Repeat the movement until the whole of the top of the shoulders has been covered.

> *key note*
>
> This technique loosens tension in the muscles across the top of the shoulders, by squeezing the toxins from the muscles and mobilising the tissues.

10. FINGER PULLS across the top of the shoulders

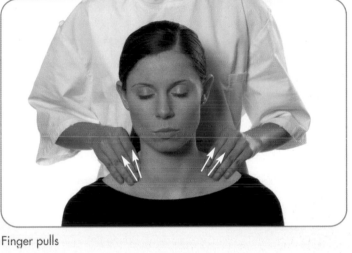

Finger pulls

Therapist's stance

Standing behind the client, in a walk standing position.

Technique

- Place both hands over the top of the shoulders, with the thumbs anchored across the back and the fingers in front of the shoulders.
- Draw the muscles in between your fingers and thumbs and lift upwards and back towards you.
- Repeat several times, until the whole of the top of the shoulder has been thoroughly covered.

> *key note*
>
> This technique helps to squeeze the toxins from the muscle fibres and encourage fresh oxygen and nutrients into the muscles. It also helps to soften and loosen the muscles, thereby easing tension.

11. SQUEEZING AND RELEASING across the top of the shoulders

Therapist's stance

Standing behind the client, in a walk standing position.

Technique

- Place palms of both hands on the top of the shoulders, with the heel of the hand lying on the trapezius muscle and fingers resting on the front of the shoulder.

- Lift and squeeze the muscles in an upwards motion with the heel of the hands and the fingers, clasping the muscles tightly in the palms of the hands.
- Squeeze using medium pressure and hold for a few seconds before releasing.
- Move further in towards the neck and repeat until the area across the top of the shoulders has been covered.

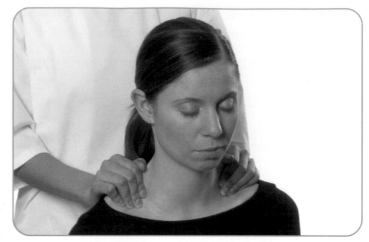

Squeezing and releasing

key note

This technique helps to squeeze and release toxins from the muscles, as well as softening and loosening tight muscle fibres.

12. HEEL PUSHES across the top of the shoulders

Therapist's stance

Standing behind the client, in a walk standing position.

Technique

- Place palms of both hands on the top of the shoulders, with the heel of the hand lying on the trapezius muscle and fingers resting on the front of the shoulder.

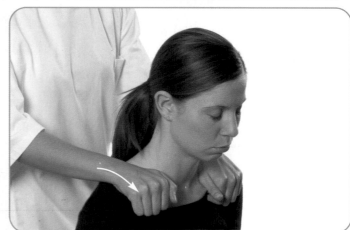

Heel pushes

- Lift up and squeeze the muscles in an upwards motion and then roll the hands forwards across to the front of the shoulders, slowly releasing the muscle from your hands as you go.
- Repeat several times, until the whole of the top of the shoulders has been covered.

key note

This technique helps to mobilise and loosen the muscles across the top of the shoulders, encouraging the client to release tension.

13. SMOOTHING with the forearms

Therapist's stance

Standing behind the client, in a walk standing position.

Technique

- Place the inside of the forearms across the top of your client's shoulders and gently apply pressure downwards.
- Glide the forearms across the top of the shoulders, rotating them as you proceed to the outer edge of the shoulder and down the upper arms to just above the elbow.
- Release and then brush the forearms back up the arms and onto the top of the shoulders.
- Repeat three times.

Smoothing

key note

This technique stretches and releases the muscles across the top of the shoulders and helps to encourage the drainage of toxins from the tissues. It also encourages the shoulders to release tension.

14. CHOPPING across the shoulders and upper back

Therapist's stance

Therapist's position is behind the client, kneeling down or standing up with the knees bent, depending on preference and client height.

Technique

- Place the palms of both hands across the upper back, with fingers together and fingertips pointing upwards.

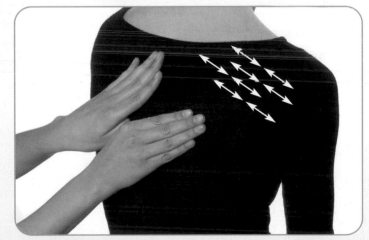

Chopping

- Perform light, brisk chopping movements by quickly moving the index fingers of both hands together, picking up and squeezing the tissue between the index fingers of both hands before releasing them.
- Work across the whole of the upper back and shoulders.

> ### *key note*
>
> This technique helps to loosen the muscles across the upper back and shoulders and stimulates the blood circulation and nerve endings, bringing about a refreshing feeling.

15. CHAMPI/DOUBLE HACKING *across the shoulders and upper back*

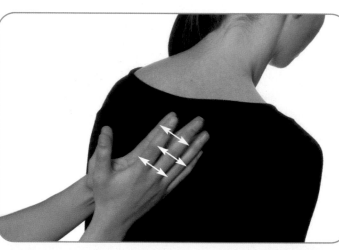

Champi

Therapist's stance

Standing behind the client, in a walk standing position.

Technique

- Hold your hands in a praying position, leaving the heels of the hands and the fingertips loosely in contact.
- Relax the hands and wrists.
- Using the tips of both fingers, joined like a cage, to strike the surface lightly and then spring off again.
- Start on one side of the spine of the upper back, around the shoulders and then back down again.
- Repeat on the other side.

NB. Take care to ensure that hacking is not performed directly over the spine.

> ### *key note*
>
> This technique stimulates the nerve endings and blood circulation, giving a refreshing and revitalising feeling.

16. SQUEEZING AND RELEASING *across the top of the shoulders (repeated as in 11)*

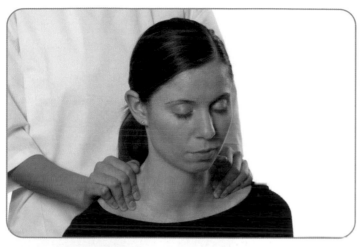

Squeezing and releasing

17. SMOOTHING *(as Step 3)*

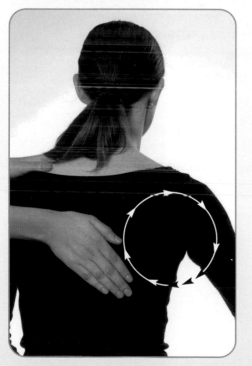

Effleurage/smoothing

18. HOLDING POSITION *(as Step 2)*

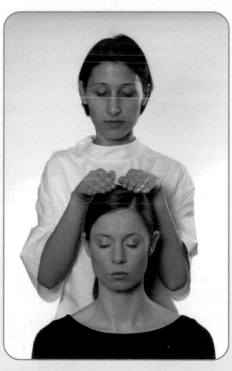

Holding position

Upper arms

The upper arms are important for upper body movement and when the shoulders are tense they tighten and restrict movement. When in a state of tension, the upper arms tend to hug the chest either at the sides or in front, while the elbows bend up.

> ## *key note*
>
> Indian Head Massage can help to reduce tension and tightness in the upper arm muscles, to help improve flexibility of the arms and shoulders.

1. SQUEEZING AND RELEASING the upper arms

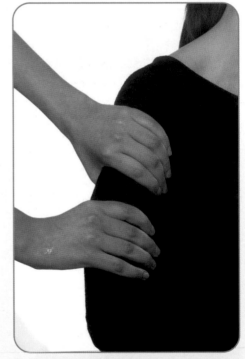

Therapist's stance

Therapist stands to the side of the client, standing behind the upper arms.

Technique

- Stand to one side of your client, behind the upper arm.
- Place the palms of both hands (one above the other) around the upper arm (thumbs resting towards the back of the upper arm and fingertips resting towards the front).
- Starting at the top, gently squeeze and release the upper arm muscles by pressing the fingers towards the thumbs, and then slowly releasing.
- Continue working down the upper arm, towards the elbow.
- Stroke lightly back up to the top of the upper arm, and repeat three times.
- Then lightly brush across the top of the client's shoulders to repeat the movement on the client's other arm.

Squeezing and releasing

> ## *key note*
>
> This technique helps loosen tension in the upper arms.

2. COMPRESSION of the upper arms

Therapist's stance

Therapist stands to the side of the client, standing behind the upper arm.

Technique

- Stand to face your client's upper arm.
- With fingers facing towards the floor, place one palm on the front of the upper arm and one on the back.
- Starting from the top of the upper arm, use the palms of both hands to compress towards one another gently, to squeeze the muscles of the upper arm.
- Slowly release and then continue working down the upper arm until you reach the elbow.
- Brush lightly back up to the top and repeat two times.

> **key note**
>
> This technique helps to encourage lymphatic drainage by squeezing toxins from the tissues of the upper arms.

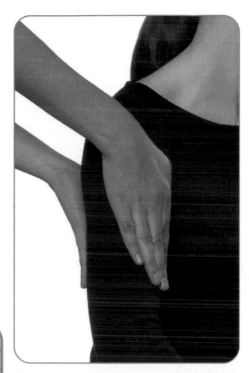

Compression

3. HEEL ROLLS embracing the upper arms

Therapist's stance

Standing behind the client, in a walk standing position.

Technique

- Place your hands facing forwards, on top of the deltoid muscles, heels of the hands behind.
- Roll the heels of your hands over the muscles of the upper arms until they reach your fingertips.
- Repeat at the middle of the upper arms and just above the elbow.

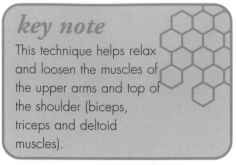

key note

This technique helps relax and loosen the muscles of the upper arms and top of the shoulder (biceps, triceps and deltoid muscles).

4. SQUEEZING AND KNEADING down the upper arms

Therapist's stance

Standing behind the client, in a walk standing position.

Technique

- Cup the hands around the cap of the shoulder, thumbs pointing forwards and fingertips behind.
- Draw your hands from under the back of the client's upper arms and squeeze up and round towards the front of the upper arms.
- Repeat this movement down to the elbows and then sweep back up to the cap of the shoulder, and repeat.

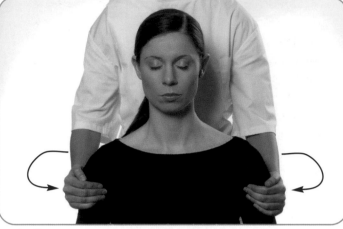

Heel rolls

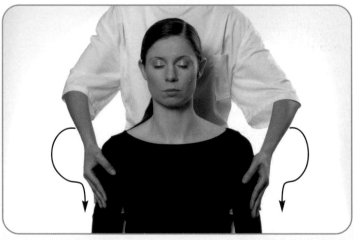

Squeezing and kneading

key note

This technique mobilises the muscles of the upper arms and helps to release tension.

5. SHOULDER MOBILISATION

Therapist's stance

Therapist stands to one side of the client, facing the shoulder and upper arm.

Technique

- Stand to one side of your client.

- Place one hand on the top of the client's shoulder and one hand under the elbow, supporting your client's hand in the crook of your elbow.
- Gently mobilise the shoulder in clockwise and anti-clockwise directions, taking the shoulder through its full range of movement.
- Repeat on the other side.

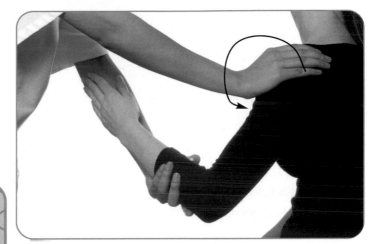

Shoulder mobilisation

key note

This technique encourages joint mobility and helps to release tension and restrictions in the shoulder joint.

6. SHOULDER LIFT

Therapist's stance

Therapist stands behind the client and bends knees.

Technique

- Ask your client to place their hands on their lap.
- Place your hands under their elbows and ask the client to take in a long, deep breath.
- As they breathe in, pull the shoulder up and outwards.
- On the client's out breath, release the shoulders back down.
- Repeat two times.

key note

This technique symbolises letting tension go and helps the client to drop their shoulders and release the tension.

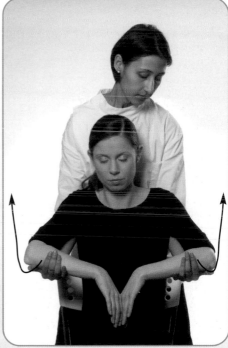

Shoulder lift

7. EFFLEURAGE/SMOOTHING WITH THE FOREARMS *down the upper arms*

Therapist's stance
Standing behind the client, in a walk standing position.

Technique
- Using the inside of the forearms, apply gentle pressure on both sides across the top of the shoulders.
- Glide the forearms across the top of the shoulders, rotating them as you proceed to the outer edge of the shoulder and down the upper arms to just above the elbow.
- Release and then brush the forearms back up the arms.
- Repeat three times.

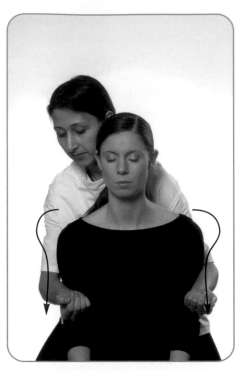

Effleurage/smoothing

The neck

When the body is balanced, the neck is designed to allow the head to move in a variety of directions. When the body is out of balance and under stress, the head tends to come forwards and the chin juts out. This then throws the body out of alignment as the neck muscles tense and take the weight of the head. The neck muscles are then in a permanent state of contraction and can cause the neck to become stiff and tight. The tension then reduces mobility of the neck and shoulders.

> ### *key note*
> Working on the neck with Indian Head Massage helps to open up the energy flow from the spine to the whole head and can help to reduce tension and improve posture by re-aligning the muscles, thereby increasing mobility and allowing the head to move more freely.

Health and safety note: During the neck massage it is important to support the client's head fully in order to avoid neck strain.

Neck massage

1. ROCKING the head backwards and forwards

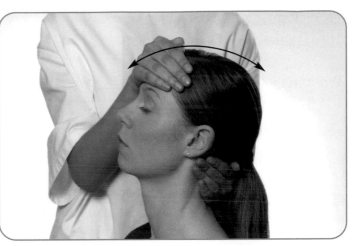

Rocking the head

Therapist's stance

Therapist stands to the side of the client.

Technique

- Place one hand on the forehead and one hand at the back of the neck.
- Ask your client to drop the head slightly forwards so you can support its weight.
- Gently rock the head forwards and backwards, taking care to avoid hyperextending the neck.
- If the neck appears tight, ask the client to breathe deeply three times to relax, after which the head should move more freely and with less resistance.

key note

This technique helps the therapist to assess how much tension there is in the neck and can help the client to relax the neck muscles.

2. SQUEEZE AND RELEASE the muscles at the back of the neck

Therapist's stance

Therapist stands to the side of the client.

Technique

- Place one hand on the client's forehead.
- Ask your client to tip their head back slightly.
- Spread your thumbs and fingers of the other hand either side of the base of the neck (forming a V shape).
- Using firm contact with the skin, slide your hand in to squeeze and lift the muscles of the back of the neck and then release by pulling the hand backwards.
- Start from the bottom of the neck and gradually work upwards until you reach the base of the skull.

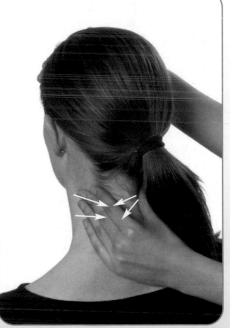

Squeeze and release

> ## key note
>
> This technique helps release tension that builds up in the back of the neck and the skull.

3. FINGER FRICTIONS to the top of the shoulders and up the side of the neck

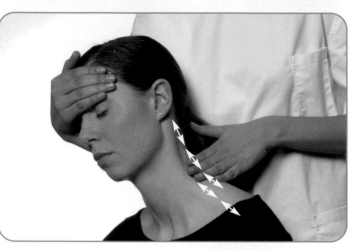

Finger frictions

Therapist's stance

Therapist stands behind the client, to one side.

Technique

- Tilt the client's head gently to one side.
- Support your client's head by using your forearm to cup around the side of their head so that it rests comfortably into your forearm.
- Perform frictions using the pads of the fingers in a side-to-side motion, across the top of the shoulder and up the side of the neck to behind the ear.
- Repeat three times.
- Repeat techniques to the other side of the neck.

> ## key note
>
> This technique helps increase the blood and lymph supply to the neck. It also builds up heat in the muscles from the frictions and helps to relieve tightness in the muscles at the side of the neck.

4. THUMB PUSHES to the side of the neck

Therapist's stance

Therapist stands behind the client, to one side.

Technique

- Retain the same support for the client's head as in technique 3.
- Use the thumb to push deeply into the muscles of the neck by pushing forwards horizontally across from the back of the neck, to the side of the neck just below the ears.

- Repeat techniques to the other side of the neck.

NB: Caution is necessary during this technique, in order to avoid applying pressure to the carotid arteries at the side of the neck and to respiratory structures such as the trachea on the front of the neck.

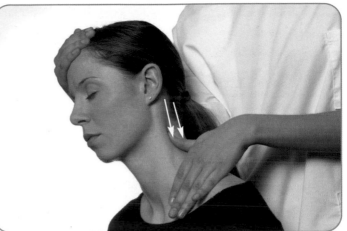

Thumb pushes

key note

This technique helps to break down fibrous adhesions that restrict movements of the head and neck.

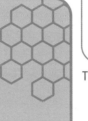

5. SQUEEZING AND RELEASING at the side of the neck

Therapist's stance

Therapist stands behind the client, to one side.

Technique

- Retain the same support for the head as in technique 3.
- Form a V shape between the thumb and the forefinger (thumb is anchored at the back).
- Squeeze and release the muscles at the side of the neck by lifting the tissue and pulling the forefinger back towards the thumb.
- Start from the side of the neck and work from the bottom upwards to up behind the ears.
- Repeat to the other side of the neck.

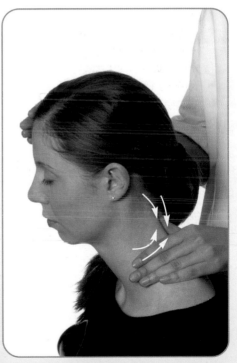

Squeezing and releasing

key note

This technique helps to squeeze the toxins from the muscles and encourages lymph drainage to the neck.

6. FINGER FRICTIONS *to the base of the skull*

Therapist's stance

Therapist stands to one side of the client.

Technique

- Support the client's forehead with one hand.
- Use your other hand to perform frictions with the pads of the fingers up and down the back of the neck.
- Work from the base of the neck to the base of the skull.
- Repeat until the back of the neck and skull have been covered.

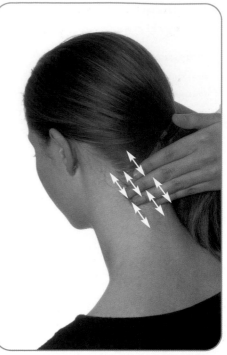

Finger frictions

> ### key note
>
> This technique helps encourage heat to release tight congested muscles at the back of the neck and the base of the skull, where tension builds up.

7. HEEL OF THE HAND FRICTIONS *to the base of the skull*

Therapist's stance

Therapist stands to one side of the client.

Technique

- Retaining the supporting hand on the forehead, use the heel of the other hand to apply friction at the base of the skull.

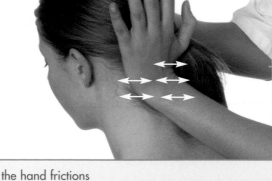

Heel of the hand frictions

- Mould the heel of the hand to the base of the skull and use a side-to-side motion to friction briskly across the base of the skull.
- Repeat until the whole area of the base of the skull has been covered.

> ### key note
>
> This technique helps to encourage the release of toxins from tight congested muscles at the base of the skull.

8. EFFLEURAGE/ SMOOTHING to the back of the neck

Therapist's stance

Therapist stands to one side of the client.

Technique

- Still retaining the supporting hand across the forehead, use the other hand to smooth the base of the skull and neck in a circular motion.
- Repeat several times.

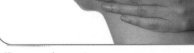

Effleurage/smoothing

key note

This technique helps to relax and soothe the neck muscles.

9. PRESSURE POINTS at the base of the skull

Therapist's stance

Therapist stands to one side of the client.

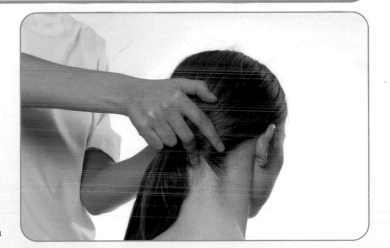

Pressure points

Technique

- Keep the supporting hand across the front of the head.
- Use the tip of the middle finger to press gently into the pressure point in the centre of the base of the skull for a few seconds, while at the same time gently rocking the head backwards.
- Pause for a second and then move the head forwards to release.
- Then use the thumb and the middle finger to press on the points approximately one inch either side of the central point, and rock the head gently backwards.
- Pause and then move the head forwards to release.

key note

This technique helps to relieve pressure from congested nerves and muscles relating to the head and neck.

10. GENTLE STRETCHING
to the side of the neck

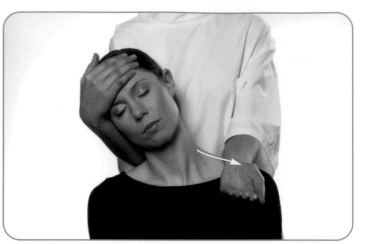

Gentle stretching

Therapist's stance

Therapist stands behind the client, to one side.

Technique

- Tilt your client's head gently to one side.
- Support your client's head by using your forearm to cup around the side of their head, so that it rests comfortably into the forearm.
- Place your other forearm on top of the client's shoulder.
- Ask your client to take a deep breath in and as they breathe out gently press down on the top of the shoulder and hold for a few seconds before sweeping down and over the top of the upper arm.
- Repeat two times.
- Then repeat the technique on the other side of the neck.

> *key note*
>
> This technique creates a gentle stretch up the side of the neck.

11. SMOOTHING WITH THE WHOLE HAND at the base of the skull (repeated as in 8)

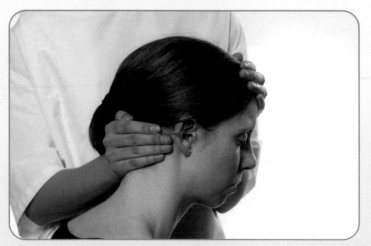

Smoothing with the whole hand

The scalp

The scalp muscles tighten when under stress, restricting the blood flow and leading to headaches, eyestrain, and neck and shoulder tension.

> ### key note
> Indian Head Massage helps to counterbalance stress in the head by improving the circulation and the condition of the hair. Regular head massage also helps to relax the muscles and nerve fibres of the scalp, thereby relieving tension and fatigue.

Scalp massage

1. RUBBING to the side of the scalp, around the ears

Therapist's stance

Therapist stands behind the client.

Technique

- Support one side of the head with one hand.
- Use the fleshy part of the palm of the other hand to carry out a light rubbing movement with side-to-side motion, across the temporalis muscle above, in front of and behind the ears.
- Work backwards and forwards three times.
- Repeat to other side.

> ### key note
> This technique helps lightly to increase the circulation of blood to the scalp.

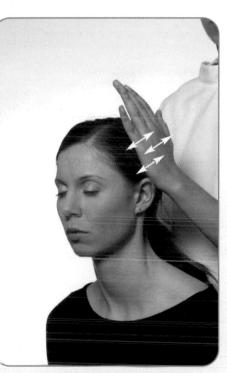

Rubbing to the side of the scalp

2. FRICTIONS *to the side of the scalp, around the ears*

Therapist's stance

Therapist stands behind the client.

Technique

- Support one side of the head with one hand.
- Use the pad of the fingers of the other hand to perform frictions briskly to the same area as the previous technique.
- Repeat on the other side of the scalp.

> ### *key note*
> This technique helps to loosen tension from the temporalis muscle that can cause headaches.

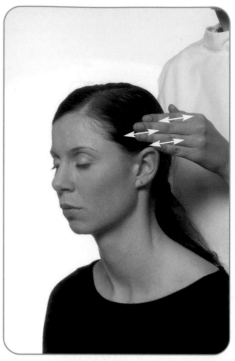

Frictions

3. RUBBING *to the whole of the scalp*

Therapist's stance

Therapist stands behind the client.

Technique

- Support one side of the client's head with one hand.
- Use the soft fleshy part of other hand to carry out rubbing motion using a broad zig-zag motion from side to side.
- Work over one side of the head from front to back and then repeat on the other side.

> ### *key note*
> This technique helps to loosen up tight scalp muscles and encourages blood and lymph supply to the scalp.

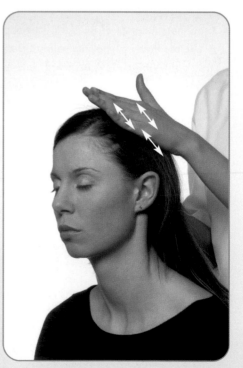

Rubbing

4. FRICTIONS with the whole of the hand

Therapist's stance

Therapist stands behind the client.

Technique

- Support one side of your client's head.
- Apply firm pressure using the whole hand in a side-to-side zig-zag motion, moving the scalp up and down.
- Work over one side of the scalp, from the front of the scalp to the back.
- Repeat to the other side.

> ### key note
> This technique increases the circulation to the scalp and loosens tight scalp muscles.

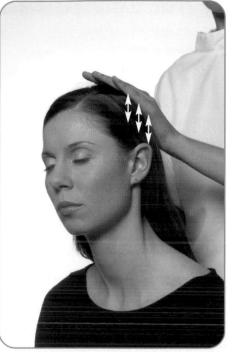

Frictions with whole hand

5. RUFFLING through the hair

Therapist's stance

Therapist stands behind the client.

Technique

- Support one side of the client's head with one hand.
- Separate the fingers of the other hand and use the tips of the fingers to perform a light wave-like movement from side to side through the hair.
- Work from the front of the scalp towards the back.
- Repeat three times.

> ### key note
> This technique has a very soothing and soporific effect on the nerves if performed slowly and is more stimulating and invigorating if performed more vigorously.

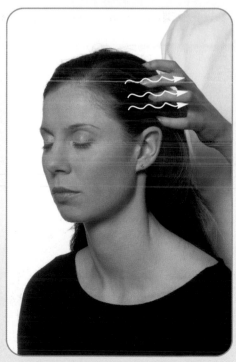

Ruffling

6. HAIR TUGGING

Therapist's stance

Therapist stands behind the client.

Technique

- Draw the fingers of both hands through the client's hair, from root to tip, in an upwards direction.
- Release the hair from your fingers, repeating several times.
- Then gather the hair between your fingers and give the hair a tug to stimulate its growth.

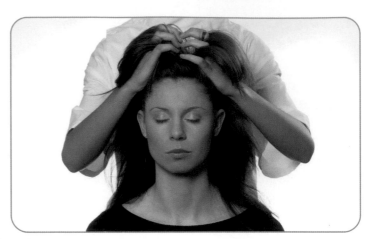

Hair tugging

key note

This technique helps to stimulate the circulation to the scalp and helps to bring fresh blood and lymph to the surface.

7. EFFLEURAGE/ SMOOTHING through the hair

Therapist's stance

Therapist stands behind the client.

Technique

- With alternate hands, stroke through the hair using the fingertips.
- Work repetitively from the front of the scalp towards the back, several times.
- If your client requires more stimulation to the scalp, use nails of both hands to comb through the hair from front to back.

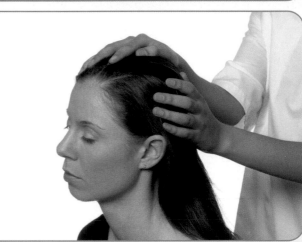

Effleurage/smoothing

key note

This technique has a very calming and soothing effect on the client.

8. TABLA PLAYING over the scalp

Therapist's stance

Therapist stands behind the client.

Technique

- Use the fingertips of both hands to perform a light drumming motion over the head.
- Work from the front of the head towards the back.

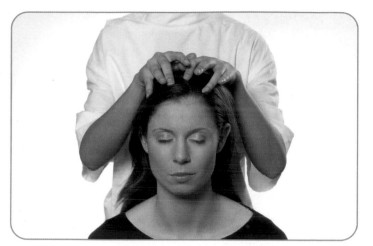

Tabla playing

key note

This technique is very stimulating and energising to the scalp.

9. PRESSURE POINTS over the scalp

Therapist's stance

Therapist stands behind the client.

Technique

- Support one side of the client's head.
- With the other hand, use the tips of all the fingers and the thumb to perform pressures (with a pumping action) across the scalp, at approximately one-inch intervals.
- Work from the hairline towards the back of the head.
- Use the fingers and thumb to press in slowly for a couple of seconds and then release.
- Work across from one side of the head to the other, changing the supporting hand when you reach the centre of the scalp.

key note

This technique helps to release blockages from the nerves relating to the head and neck and has a stimulating effect on the head.

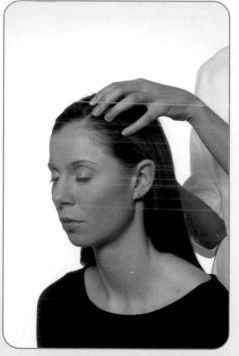

Pressure points

10. SQUEEZE AND RELEASE the scalp muscles

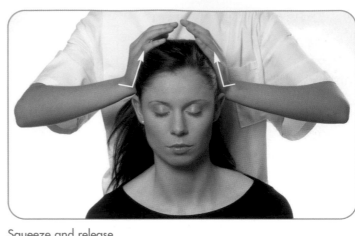

Squeeze and release

Therapist's stance

Therapist stands behind the client.

Technique

- Place your fingers on top of the client's head, with the heels of the hands placed behind the ears.
- Squeeze inwards with medium pressure with the heels of the hands.
- Hold and then lift and release upwards.
- Repeat the movement with the heels of hands above the ears.
- Repeat the movement with the hands placed in front of the ears.

key note

This technique helps to relieve headaches and eyestrain.

11. CIRCULAR FRICTIONS using the heels of the hands across the temples

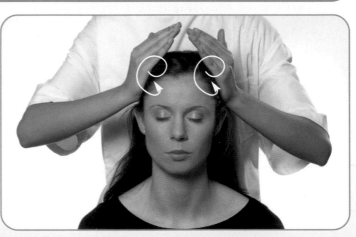

Circular frictions

Therapist's stance

Therapist stands behind the client.

Technique

- Support the client's head against you.
- Use the heels of both hands to make circular movements against the temples.
- Lift upwards and back towards you.
- Repeat several times.

key note

This technique is also very effective at helping to relieve tension headaches and eyestrain.

12. COMPRESSION to the head

Therapist's stance

Therapist stands to the side of the client.

Technique

- Place one hand round the front of the head and one round the back.
- Squeeze inwards with the palms of the hands and then release.
- Repeat three times.

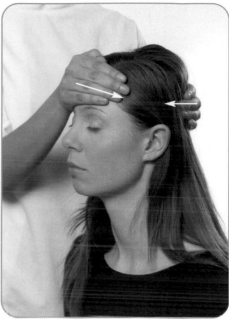

Compression

> **key note**
>
> This technique is very effective at helping to release tension headaches.

13. EFFLEURAGE/ SMOOTHING through the hair (repeated as in 7)

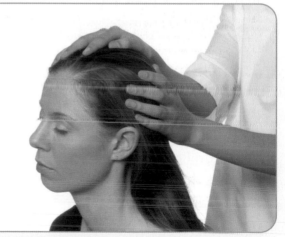

Effleurage/smoothing

The face

The face is an area of the body that cannot help but show tension. When a person is feeling tense the jaw tends to clamp tight, teeth grind together and the lips tighten.

> **key note**
>
> Indian Head Massage can help to relax the facial muscles and melt away tension, leaving the client feeling calm and refreshed.

Before commencing the face massage, you may wish to use a dry hand cleanser to cleanse your hands of any oil or sebum that may be left on the hands from the scalp massage.

For the face massage, the client's head needs to be tilted back slightly to rest against the therapist's upper thorax. Ensure that the client's neck is comfortable and offer a neck support or cushion.

1. EFFLEURAGE/ SMOOTHING across the face

Therapist's stance
Therapist stands behind the client.

Technique
- Start with the fingers across the chin.
- Use the fingers of both hands to smooth the face with gentle flowing movements in an upwards direction.
- Work across the chin and jaw, then across cheeks and across the forehead.
- Repeat three times.

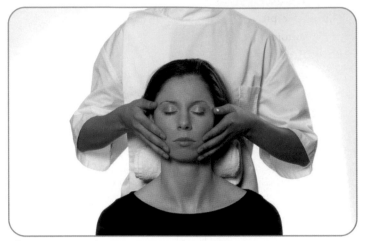
Effleurage/smoothing

key note
This technique helps to relax and soothe tired facial muscles.

2. PRESSURE POINTS across the forehead, around the eye sockets and cheek- bones

Therapist's stance
Therapist stands behind the client.

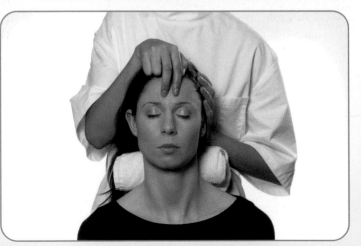
Pressure points

Technique
- Support the client's head with one hand
  - **a** use the pads of the forefinger and middle finger of the other hand
    to press the following pressure points in pairs at the midline of the forehead.
    - ▸ Pair 1: half an inch above the bridge of the nose

▸ Pair 2: halfway up the forehead
▸ Pair 3: at the hairline.
- Then move both fingers outwards approximately half an inch and repeat

b Then press points on ridge of bone all round the eyes – outwards along the top and inwards along the bottom.

c Now move to points either side of nose and across the curve of the cheekbones and drain sinuses by curving forefingers under cheekbones and holding for a few seconds.

> *key note*
>
> This technique helps to relieve sinus congestion and encourage lymphatic drainage from the head.

3. CIRCULAR TEMPLE FRICTIONS with the tips of the fingers

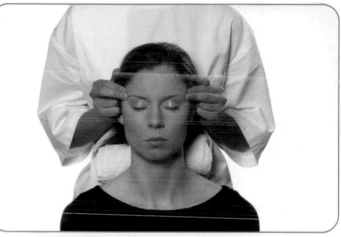

Circular temple frictions

Therapist's stance
Therapist stands behind the client.

Technique
- Support the client's head against you.
- Use the pads of the fingers to perform circular frictions to the temples.
- Work slowly and deeply over the area several times.

> *key note*
>
> This technique helps to relieve tension in facial muscles, relieves headaches and eyestrain and helps to relax the eyes.

4. SQUEEZING AND TWIDDLING the ear lobes

Therapist's stance
Therapist stands behind client.

Technique
- Place your fingers behind the client's ear lobes and the thumbs in front.

- Squeeze the ear lobes in between thumb and forefinger.
- Hold for a few seconds and then slowly release.
- Then twiddle the ears by rolling the thumb and the forefinger across the ear lobe in a brisk manner.
- Repeat several times.

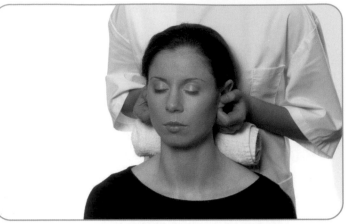

Squeezing and twiddling ear lobes

key note

This technique stimulates the nerve endings to the whole of the body and creates an energising feeling.

5. EFFLEURAGE/SMOOTHING (as in 1)

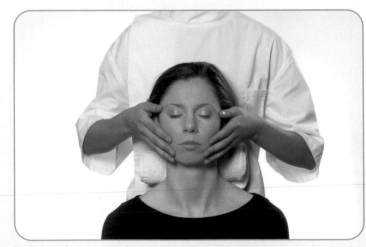

Effleurage/smoothing

6. RELAXING the facial muscles

Therapist's stance

Therapist stands behind the client.

Technique

- Gently place both of your hands so that they cover the lower part of the jaw and cheeks.

- Relax the hands and keep them still and relaxed for a few seconds.
- Gradually move the hands up the face, stopping to place the hands so that the tips of the middle fingers meet at the bridge of the nose.
- Continue up the face, stopping to place the hands so that they cover the eyes.
- Continue up the face, finally placing hands over the top of the forehead.

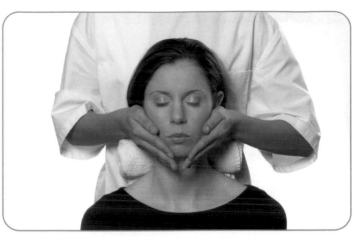

Relaxing facial muscles

key note

This technique relaxes the facial muscles and the eyes, and creates a feeling of stillness and calm.

7. HIGHER CHAKRA BALANCING

Therapist's stance

Therapist stands to the side of the client.

Technique

- Place one hand lightly over the crown chakra (top of the client's head) and cup the other hand over the throat chakra (without touching the throat).
- Hold your hands there for a short while, breathing deeply and slowly to concentrate.
- Retaining the hand over the crown chakra, move the other hand up to place lightly over the third eye, and hold there for a few moments.
- Then place both hands over the crown.

key note

Chakra balancing helps to re-align the client's energy and is very soothing and calming, helping to bring about a sense of peace and harmony.

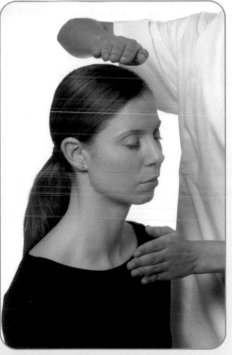

Higher chakra balancing

8. *SQUEEZE AND RELEASE the back of the neck*

Therapist's stance
Therapist stands to the side of the client.

Technique
- Place one hand over the third eye area of the client's forehead.
- Spread the thumbs and fingers of your other hand either side of the base of the neck (forming a V shape) and gently squeeze and release the muscles at the back of the neck.

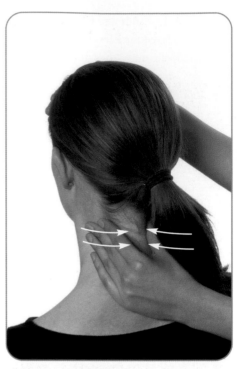

Squeeze and release

9. *EFFLEURAGE/SMOOTHING across the upper back*

This helps to get the client grounded and bring them back from a deep state of relaxation.

10. *SLOWLY LEAVE THE CLIENT'S AURA*

After squeezing the top of the shoulders, take a step back from the client's aura and gently shake your hands.

Wash your hands.

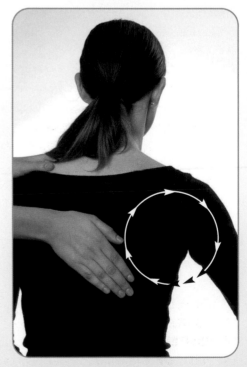

Effleurage/smoothing

Full Routine Quick Reference Guide

Upper back and shoulder massage

1 **STARTING POSITION** with hands over the top of the client's shoulders
2 **HOLDING POSITION** over the top of the head
3 **EFFLEURAGE/SMOOTHING** across the shoulders and upper back
4 **PETRISSAGE/THUMB SWEEPING** across the shoulders
5 **FRICTIONS WITH THE HEEL OF THE HAND** rubbing around the scapulae
6 **FRICTIONS WITH THE FINGER** rubbing around the scapulae
7 **SMOOTHING EFFLEURAGE** (repeated us in 3)
8 **PRESSURES** with the knuckles either side of the spine
9 **THUMB PUSHES** over the shoulders
10 **FINGER PULLS** across the top of the shoulders
11 **SQUEEZING AND RELEASING** across the top of the shoulders
12 **HEEL PUSHES** across the top of the shoulders
13 **SMOOTHING** with the forearms
14 **CHOPPING** across the shoulders and upper back
15 **CHAMPI/DOUBLE HACKING** across the shoulders and upper back
16 **SQUEEZING AND RELEASING** across the top of the shoulders (repeated as in 11)
17 **SMOOTHING** (repeated as in 3)
18 **HOLDING POSITION** over the tops of the shoulders (repeated as in 2)

Upper arms

1 **SQUEEZING AND RELEASING** the upper arms
2 **COMPRESSION** of the upper arms
3 **HEEL ROLLS** embracing the upper arms
4 **SQUEEZING AND KNEADING** down the upper arms
5 **GENTLE MOBILISATION** of the shoulders
6 **SHOULDER LIFT**
7 **SMOOTHING WITH THE FOREARMS** down the upper arms

The neck

1 **ROCKING** the head backwards and forwards
2 **SQUEEZE AND RELEASE** the muscles at the back of the neck
3 **FINGER FRICTIONS** to the top of the shoulders and up the side of the neck
4 **THUMB PUSHES** to the side of the neck
5 **SQUEEZING AND RELEASING** at the side of the neck
6 **FINGER FRICTIONS** to the base of the skull
7 **HEEL OF THE HAND FRICTIONS** to the base of the skull
8 **SMOOTHING WITH THE WHOLE HAND** at the base of the skull

9 **PRESSURE POINTS** at the base of the skull

10 **GENTLE STRETCHING** to the side of the neck

11 **SMOOTHING WITH THE WHOLE HAND** at the base of the skull (repeated as in 8)

The scalp

1 **RUBBING** to the side of the scalp, around the ears

2 **FRICTIONS** to the side of the scalp, around the ears

3 **RUBBING** to the whole of the scalp

4 **WHOLE OF THE HAND FRICTIONS** to the whole of the scalp

5 **RUFFLING** through the hair

6 **TUGGING/PLUCKING WITH THE FINGERS** through the hair

7 **SMOOTHING WITH THE FINGERTIPS** through the hair

8 **TAPPING** over the scalp

9 **PRESSURE POINTS** over the scalp

10 **SQUEEZING** the scalp muscles

11 **CIRCULAR FRICTIONS USING THE HEELS OF THE HANDS** across the temples

12 **COMPRESSION** to the head

13 **FINISH BY SMOOTHING WITH THE FINGERTIPS** through the hair (repeated as in 7)

The face

1 **SMOOTHING** across the face

2 **PRESSURE POINTS** across the forehead, around the eye sockets and cheekbones

3 **CIRCULAR TEMPLE FRICTIONS** with the tips of the fingers

4 **SQUEEZING AND TWIDDLING** the ear lobes

5 **SMOOTHING** (repeated as in 1)

6 **RELAXING** the facial muscles

7 **HIGHER CHAKRA BALANCING**

8 **GENTLE SQUEEZE AND RELEASE** to the back of the neck

9 **GENTLY SMOOTH** across the upper back

10 **SLOWLY LEAVE THE CLIENT'S AURA**

After-Care Advice

Clients will often feel deeply relaxed following treatment. It is therefore important that they have a suitable rest period and are offered a glass of water before rising.

If oil has been used on the scalp, then clients should be encouraged to leave the oil on for a few hours after treatment before shampooing. When washing their hair after oil application, clients should be advised not to wet their hair first but to apply shampoo to the scalp before the water in order to help emulsify the oil.

As part of a client's home care programme, therapists may wish to teach clients simple self-massage techniques for the scalp with oils, particularly if the client requires an improvement to their hair condition.

In order to aid the healing process and to get the maximum benefit from their treatments, clients are advised to:

- increase intake of water following treatment, to assist the body's detoxification process
- have a suitable rest period after the treatment
- avoid eating a heavy meal after the treatment; try to keep the diet light while the body is using its energy for healing
- avoid smoking
- cut down on consumption of stimulants such as tea, coffee, alcohol and drugs
- take time out to relax and practise stress-relieving techniques such as yoga or meditation, if appropriate
- participate in regular manageable exercise
- practise the correct breathing techniques to create a feeling of calm
- use oils and simple head massage techniques at home for long-term hair care

Reactions to Indian Head Massage

A client's reaction to Indian Head Massage may vary according to their physical and emotional condition. If the body has been under a considerable amount of stress, it is not unusual for there to be some kind of reaction as the body adjusts itself back to balance. This is often referred to as a 'healing crisis'. Clients should be made aware of the fact that some of these reactions may occur and be reassured that if they do occur, they will only be temporary as the body adjusts itself back to balance.

Discussed below are some of the healing reactions that may occur following an Indian Head Massage treatment:

- feeling of tiredness and lethargy because of the release of toxins
- feeling of dizziness or nausea
- aching and soreness in the muscles because of the release of toxins and the nerve fibres responding to the massage
- heightened emotional state – depression, weepiness or laughter
- increased urination
- increased secretions of mucus from the nose and mouth
- cold-like symptoms
- disturbed sleep pattern (restlessness).

Many clients report the following positive reactions following an Indian Head Massage:

- relief from stress and muscular tension
- an increased feeling of awareness; clients often experience a feeling of calm, peace and tranquillity because of the re-balancing of the chakras

- improved sleep pattern (deep and restful)
- feeling of alertness and being clearer in mental thought
- increased energy levels
- elevation of mood
- pain relief
- increased joint mobility.

Important information to be recorded after the treatment includes:

- an assessment of the client's physical condition (noting any areas of tension, physiological responses) as well as psychological responses
- visual assessment of the client (noting posture, non-verbal signs)
- any known reactions, their effects and any advice given
- after-care advice
- home care advice, along with any oils or products suggested for home use
- outcome and general evaluation of the treatment
- recommendations for future treatment and the suggested frequency.

Frequency of treatment

In India, head massage is often part of a daily schedule. In the Western world, as part of a stress management programme, Indian Head Massage should ideally be carried out once or even twice a week for maximum benefit. It is advisable to offer clients a course of treatments (between four and six initially) and to recommend that the client takes the treatments close together to start with.

Frequency of treatment may vary with a client's resources, namely time and money, and clients should be encouraged to attend for treatments as frequently as their schedule and financial resources will allow.

Benefits of regular Indian Head Massage treatments

In order to maximise the benefits of Indian Head Massage, it is important for clients to receive regular treatment.

Benefits of regular treatment include:

- improvement in hair condition
- reduction in stress levels
- increased energy levels
- a general sense of wellbeing
- improved sleep patterns
- improvement in circulation.

SELF-ASSESSMENT QUESTIONS

1 Friction movements are used in Indian Head Massage to

    a prepare the area for deeper strokes

    b stimulate and clear nerve pathways

    c break down tension nodules caused by stress and tension

    d restore energy balance to the body.

2 A form of tapotement used in Indian Head Massage called 'double hacking' is also known traditionally as

    a tabla playing

    b tapping

    c cupping

    d champi.

3 Which of the following is **not** considered to be a form of petrissage?

    a picking up

    b squeezing and releasing

    c smoothing

    d rolling

4 How many marma points are located in the head and neck area?

    a 107

    b 27

    c 37

    d 57.

5 Which of the following oils would not be suitable for a client with dry skin and hair?

    a sesame

    b mustard

    c olive

    d coconut.

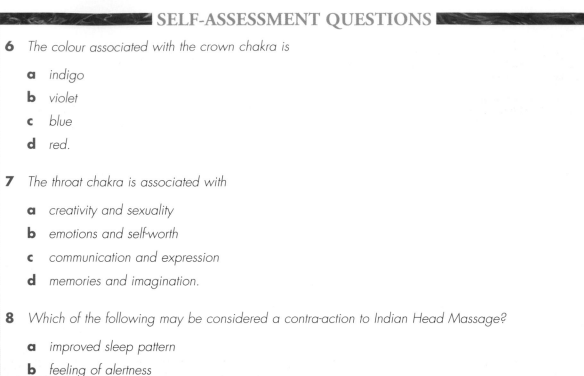

SELF-ASSESSMENT QUESTIONS

6 *The colour associated with the crown chakra is*

   a *indigo*

   b *violet*

   c *blue*

   d *red.*

7 *The throat chakra is associated with*

   a *creativity and sexuality*

   b *emotions and self-worth*

   c *communication and expression*

   d *memories and imagination.*

8 *Which of the following may be considered a contra-action to Indian Head Massage?*

   a *improved sleep pattern*

   b *feeling of alertness*

   c *headache and nausea*

   d *increased energy levels.*

Stress Management

7

Stress is a common feature of modern life and is therefore something everyone experiences. Nobody is born knowing how to handle stress and, as there is no immunity from it, the best way to protect the body from the harmful effects of stress is to learn how to manage it.

Stress undermines the state of physical and emotional well being; learning how to manage stress effectively can therefore help to maintain good health and vitality.

It is now acknowledged that many medical conditions are stress-related and therefore more importance is being placed on being able to handle stress in order to improve health.

The increase in stress levels is a major factor responsible for the increase in popularity of holistic therapies such as Indian Head Massage, as the value of stress relief and relaxation provided by treatments can be a major factor in helping clients to manage their own stress.

By the end of this chapter, you will be able to relate the following to your work in Indian Head Massage:

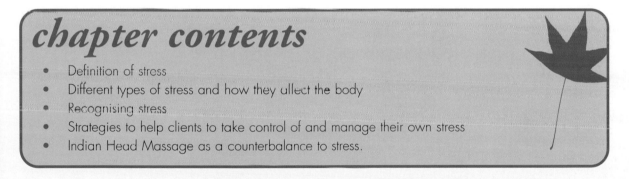

chapter contents

- Definition of stress
- Different types of stress and how they affect the body
- Recognising stress
- Strategies to help clients to take control of and manage their own stress
- Indian Head Massage as a counterbalance to stress.

By the very nature of their work, holistic therapists are exposed to a considerable amount of emotional energy when dealing with clients. It is therefore important for them to be able to use stress management techniques in order to help both their clients and themselves.

Indian Head Massage can be a very effective treatment in counterbalancing some of the negative effects of stress. However, for long-term stress relief, clients often need to consider many other factors in their life. This chapter considers the basic tools of stress management, from identifying the symptoms and causes to employing strategies for coping with stress.

Definition of Stress

There is no conclusive definition of 'stress'. It is a difficult term to define, as stress means different things to different people.

However, it can be said that stress is the adaptive response to the demands or pressures placed upon an individual, and can involve any interference that disturbs a person's emotional and physical well being. The stress becomes unacceptable when the pressures are beyond the control of the individual and the results of the stress can then be harmful to others. Stress is therefore the imbalance between the demands of everyday life and the ability to cope with them.

Stress can be positive in that it can act as a stimulus and increase levels of alertness, but it can also be negative when too much stress affects the ability to function effectively. It is the depth and number of stressors at any time that causes stress to become beyond control, which then requires the body to make adjustments to re-establish a normal balance.

Types of Stress

Survival stress

This type of stress is when the body reacts to meet the demands of a physically or emotionally threatening situation. The reaction is mediated by the release of adrenaline and produces the so-called 'fight or flight' reaction.

This type of stress is positive in that it enables the body and mind to react quickly and effectively. It is only when the effects of adrenaline are long-term that it can lead to negative stress.

Internally generated stress

This type of stress is often caused by the view of or reaction to a situation, rather than the situation itself. Anxiety and worry can lead to negative thought processes and often lead to a feeling that circumstances are out of control.

There is a relationship between personality and stress, in particular with anxious and obsessional personalities. What may be stressful for one person may be enjoyable and exciting for another.

Work/lifestyle-related stress

Many stresses that are experienced may relate to work or lifestyle. In this context, stress may come from some of the following:

*   having too much or too little work
*   time pressures and deadlines
*   demands of a job with limited resources
*   insufficient working or living space
*   disorganised working conditions
*   limited time, to the detriment of leisure and family life
*   pollution
*   financial problems
*   relationship problems

- ill health
- family situations such as a birth, death, marriage or divorce.

Negative stress

This type of stress is caused by the inability to manage long-term stress.

How to Recognise Stress

Recognising stress can be very difficult. It is important to realise that as stress levels increase, the ability to recognise stress usually decreases. Stress can manifest itself in different ways, and symptoms may be presented in a number of different ways. These are discussed below.

Short-term physical stress signals

These are symptoms of survival stress as the body adapts to situations that are perceived as a threat. Effects of short-term physical stress include an increased heart beat, rapid breathing, increased sweating, tense muscles, dry mouth, frequency of urination and feeling of nausea.

While the effects of short-term physical stress may help you survive in a threatening situation, negative stress can result when the adrenaline is not put to this use.

The effects of excess adrenaline can lead to anxiety, frustration, negative thinking, reduction in self confidence, distraction, and may cause difficult situations to be seen as a threat rather than a challenge.

Long-term stress signals

Common complaints relating to long-term stress are back pain, headaches, aches and pains, excessive tiredness, digestive problems, frequent colds, skin eruptions and exacerbation of asthma. Stress and pressure can also lead to the following:

a) INTERNAL STRESS SIGNALS

When the body is subjected to long-term stress, the mind becomes unable to think clearly and rationally about situations and problems. This can lead to feelings of anxiety, worry, confusion, feeling out of control or overwhelmed, restlessness, frustration, irritability, hostility, impatience, helplessness, depression and mood changes.

People who suffer from long-term stress may generally feel more lethargic, find difficulty sleeping, change their eating habits, rely more on medication, drink and smoke more frequently and have a reduced sex drive.

b) BEHAVIOURAL STRESS SIGNALS

When people are under pressure this can be exhibited in some of the following ways: talking too fast, twitching and fiddling, being irritable, defensive, aggressive, irritated, critical and overreacting emotionally to situations. They may also find that they start becoming more forgetful, make more mistakes, are unable to concentrate, unrealistic in their judgement and become unreasonably negative. Pressure may cause some people to neglect their personal appearance and have increasing amounts of time absent from work.

If the body is subjected to excessive short-term stress, it may lead to ineffective performance which should be treated as a warning sign; stress management strategies can be adopted to avoid the problem in the future. The effects of long-term stress, however, can be much more severe as it can lead to extreme fatigue, exhaustion, burn-out or even breakdown.

Summary of signs and symptoms of stress

1) BEHAVIOURAL CHANGES

People who suffer from stress may:

- be argumentative
- be less friendly
- become withdrawn
- avoid friends and relatives
- lose creativity
- work longer and harder and achieve less
- be reluctant to do their own job properly
- procrastinate.

2) CHANGE OF FEELINGS

People who experience stress may:

- lose their sense of humour
- have a sense of being a failure
- lack self-esteem and have a cynical and bitter attitude
- experience irritability with conflict at home and work
- feel apathetic.

3) CHANGE OF THINKING

Stress can cause people to:

- be rigid in their thinking, with resistance to change
- be suspicious
- have poor concentration
- feel like leaving a job or relationship.

4) PHYSICAL

People who are stressed may:

- feel tired all the time
- experience sleep problems (usually poor sleep)
- be increasingly absent from work because of prolonged minor illnesses

- have aches and pains
- suffer backache
- experience headaches and migraine
- have indigestion
- hyperventilate
- have palpitations.

5) **MENTAL HEALTH**

The effects of stress can cause feelings of:

- anxiety
- depression
- fear of rejection.

6) **COGNITIVE DISTORTION**

Individuals suffering from stress may view themselves in a distorted way:

- **JUMPING TO CONCLUSIONS**: even in the absence of proof, stressed individuals may jump to conclusions. They may assume that other people see them in a certain way, or they may anticipate that things will turn out badly and act as if their predictions are facts.
- **ALL OR NONE**: this is the feeling that, if you fail in one way, you see yourself as a total failure. There is then the tendency to overgeneralise and see this single failure as a proof of your life's failure.
- **MENTAL FILTER**: this is when people pick out negative events and dwell on them to the exclusion of everything else. Eventually, the positive aspects of life become rejected and ignored.

The Effects of Stress on the Body

When the body is placed under physical or psychological stress, it increases the production of certain hormones such as cortisol and adrenaline. These hormones produce marked changes in the heart rate, blood pressure levels, metabolism and physical activity. While this physical action can help a person to function more effectively when under pressure for short periods of time, it can also be extremely damaging and debilitating in the long term.

Dr Hans Selye called the body's response to stress the 'general adaptation syndrome' which he suggested be divided into three stages.

The first stage is the **alarm stage** which is the body's initial reaction to the perceived stressor. This involves the so-called 'fight or flight' syndrome which involves the sympathetic nervous system and the release of the hormones adrenaline and cortisol.

The effects on the body are to effect an alert response, and include:

- increased heart rate
- increased ventilation rate
- increased diversion of blood to the muscles and brain
- increase in perspiration

- increased release of glucose from the liver
- inhibited digestion.

The alarm stage allows the body to cope and respond and when the threat is over the body returns to a state of balance through repair and rest (parasympathetic system).

However, problems can start to occur when the restoration of balance does not happen through not allowing the body to rest sufficiently, or through perceived or real encounters with repeated stressful situations.

Repeated alarm reactions can lead to symptoms such as breathlessness, a dry mouth, aching, a clenched jaw or fists, dizziness, palpitations and sweating.

The second stage is known as the **resistance** stage which, through the secretion of the circulating hormones, allows the body to continue fighting long after the effects of the alarm reaction have dissipated. This eventually leads to symptoms of disease as the body's energy resources are drained without adequate recuperation and repair. Symptoms associated with the resistance stage include colds and flu, anxiety and depression, high blood pressure, chest pains, tiredness, insomnia, indigestion, headaches and migraine.

The third stage is the **exhaustion** stage which takes place if the stress response continues without relief and can result in organs becoming more and more compromised until the adaptation becomes degenerative.

> ### *key note*
> Increased cortisol secretion in stressful situations reduces the body's immune response and the anti-inflammatory effect of cortisol can slow down healing too.

Areas of the body most vulnerable to stress

When the body is moving or stationary, a combination of muscle tension and relaxation exists in order to maintain posture.

If a good balance is not achieved then the body suffers excessive muscle tension which can cause pain and fatigue. If muscles are held tightly in a state of contraction, circulation is impeded which results in a build-up of the products of fatigue. This can then result in muscular spasms, aches and pains.

When under stress, the entire body becomes tense and posture changes. Hours spent sitting and working at a desk can cause tension to accumulate in the upper body, particularly around the neck and shoulders. Large amounts of time spent in front of the computer screen can result in eyestrain where the eyes and surrounding muscles become tired.

Being tense and in a permanent state of alert can be uncomfortable and has the ability to throw the body out of balance. Tension uses up energy, but the energy is unproductive. Muscle tension can also affect the ability to function well as it makes our thought processes less efficient.

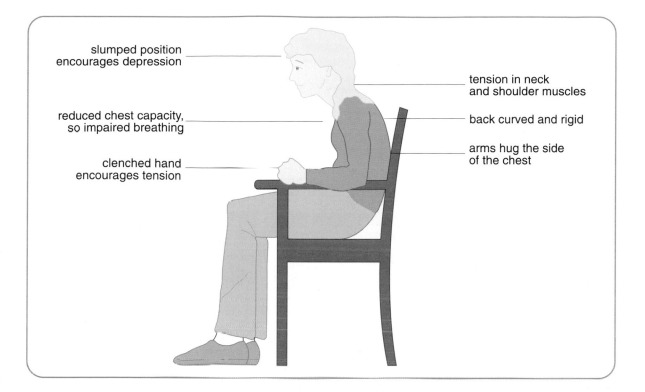

slumped position
encourages depression

tension in neck
and shoulder muscles

reduced chest capacity,
so impaired breathing

back curved and rigid

clenched hand
encourages tension

arms hug the side
of the chest

key note

Tension can also have a debilitating effect on the immune system, predisposing people to colds and other diseases, as when in a constant state of alert, it inhibits healing and tissue repair. The key to stress relief is therefore relaxation as healing can only take place when the body is at rest.

Shoulders

The shoulders are the place where most people hold a considerable amount of tension. When the body is in a state of tension the shoulders are lifted toward the ears and often remain this way causing the muscles to go into spasm. This restricts the blood flow to the head, neck and shoulders and causes the neck and shoulders to become stiff and inflexible. Sitting with hunched shoulders can reduce chest capacity and thus impair breathing.

key note

Indian Head Massage can help to counterbalance the effects of stress by relaxing the shoulders; they will then drop and allow the energy to flow more freely to the area, encouraging deeper and easier breathing and improved joint flexibility.

Upper Arms

The upper arms are important for upper body movement; when the shoulders are tense they tighten and restrict movement.

When in a state of tension, the upper arms tend to hug the chest either at the sides or in front, while the elbows bend up.

> ### *key note*
> Indian Head Massage can help reduce tension and tightness in the upper arm muscles to help improve flexibility of the arms and shoulders.

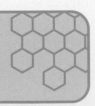

Neck

When the body is balanced the neck is designed to allow the head to move in a variety of directions. When the body is out of balance and under stress, the head tends to come forwards and the chin juts out. This then throws the body out of alignment as the neck muscles tense and take the weight of the head. The neck muscles are then in a permanent state of contraction and can cause the neck to become stiff and tight. The tension then reduces mobility of the neck and shoulders.

> ### *key note*
> Working on the neck with Indian Head Massage helps to open up the energy flow from the spine to the whole head and can help to reduce tension, improve posture by re-aligning the muscles, thereby increasing mobility and allowing the head to move more freely.

Head

The face is an area of the body that cannot help but show tension; the jaw clamps tight, teeth grind together and the lips tighten. The scalp and temporal muscles tighten when under stress, restricting the blood flow and leading to headaches, eyestrain and neck and shoulder tension.

> ### *key note*
> Indian Head Massage helps to counterbalance stress in the head by improving the circulation and relaxing the muscles and nerve fibres, thereby relieving tension.

When the body is in balance it facilitates relaxation and a positive mental outlook, which are critical to successful stress management.

If the shoulders and chest are free of tension the ribs are free to allow deep relaxed breathing; if the head and neck are well balanced they can support the shoulders and take pressure from the neck muscles.

The body is ideally equipped to deal with many different types of stressors; however, the ability to deal with stress can be inhibited by a heavy load of unresolved stress, which contributes to the development of disease and pain.

Stress-related Disorders

Stress is considered to be a contributory factor in many conditions. Listed below are areas susceptible to stress-related diseases:

- **skin** – as the skin is often a manifestation of what is felt inside, skin disorders such as eczema and psoriasis are often exacerbated by stress. Allergies may also be triggered by stress
- **hair** – some forms of hair loss are linked to stress
- **heart** – high blood pressure and conditions such as angina may be exacerbated by stress. If the blood supply to the heart is restricted by arteriosclerosis and the person's life is very stressful, a heart attack can result
- **lungs** – symptoms of asthma often worsen when the body is subjected to high levels of emotional stress
- **muscles** – muscle tension is often the result of stress
- **brain** – anxiety and depression may be triggered by stress
- **reproductive** – the reproductive hormones are reduced at times of stress; this is evidenced by stress-related problems such as infertility and menstrual disorders
- **digestion** – conditions that may be aggravated by stress include ulcers and irritable bowel syndrome.

Adaptation to Stress

Fortunately, the body has the capacity to cope with stress as the purpose of all the body's systems is to maintain a constant internal environment through homeostasis.

However, there are several factors that may affect the body's ability to deal with stress; they include the following:

- **genetics** – the effects of stress on the body can be determined by genetic make-up and can dictate how well different organs respond and adapt to stressful situations
- **physiological reserve** – the body's response to stress depends on the ability to increase or decrease function according to its needs. If the ability of an organ to respond is diminished, it is difficult for the body to maintain homeostasis; even with small demands, imbalance and disease may ensue
- **age** – with age the ability to adapt is diminished and while a young, healthy individual may respond and adapt to stress easily, an elderly client may find the situation considerably more stressful

- **health status** – clients who are mentally and physically fit are able to adapt to stress placed on them more easily than others who are not
- **nutrition** – deficiencies or excesses of nutrition can impair one's ability to adapt to stressful situations
- **sleep** – irregular sleep patterns and wakefulness can reduce immunity as well as physical and psychological functions. Sleep is important for restoring energy and if sleep is inadequate, it can impair the body's ability to deal with stress
- **psychological factors** – psychological conditions such as anxiety and depression can make a person more susceptible to stress.

Managing Stress

In order to be able to work towards prevention of stress, it is first important to be able to identify its causes.

Part of the problem with stress is its familiarity; as people become used to living with stress they may be unaware of how it is affecting them or those around them.

Mental attitude is a critical factor in dealing with stress, along with finding ways of reducing the effects of stress. Focusing on the ownership of the sources of the stress and not on the feelings they generate is the first step to counterbalancing it. Stress management can be approached in several different ways and a client's stress management programme may typically consist of experiencing a range of holistic therapies, the use of relaxation and stress reduction techniques, as well as implementing lifestyle changes.

Holistic therapists can help clients to recognise their own stress by advising on ways in which they can combat it and start to manage their own stress positively. Stress management has to take into account the recognition of an individual's vulnerability to stress, ability to be aware of possible sources of stress and identifying signs and symptoms of stress. What is most important is helping clients to learn how to manage stress, be able to identify those factors that contribute to it and so be able to control it.

Optimum stress levels

Stress levels vary, like any other human characteristic, and what may seem challenging and exciting to one person may seem stressful and threatening to another. The most positive approach to successful stress management is finding an optimum stress level in which the body can be sufficiently stimulated to perform well while not becoming overstressed and unhappy.

key note

It is important to each individual to be able to monitor their own stress levels. Some people may operate most effectively at a low level of stress, while this may leave another person feeling bored or unmotivated. Alternatively, someone who performs only moderately at low level may find they excel at a high level when they are under more pressure.

The most effective way of finding an optimum level of stress is to keep a stress diary for a short period of time, in order to be able to analyse what is causing the stress and whether it is being controlled effectively. The type of information that could be recorded in a stress diary is the stressful event and time, how stressful the event was (on a scale of 1 to 10) what made the event stressful and how the situation was handled. This can be the key to identifying whether it was the cause that was tackled or the symptom.

When analysing a stress diary, it should be possible to project the following information:

- the level of stress that is optimum for an individual
- the main sources of unpleasant or negative stress and whether the strategies for managing them are effective or not.

Managing Stress Effectively

Once there is an understanding or recognition as to what is causing the stress and the level under which an individual can work effectively, the next stage is to work out how to manage the stress. An action plan for managing stress may include:

- controlling or eliminating the problems that are causing the stress
- using stress reduction techniques
- making lifestyle changes
- taking a holiday or break more often
- social and family support
- time management
- hobbies and leisure time
- being prepared to ask for help
- looking back at action taken and evaluating the effects.

Stress reduction techniques

When choosing methods for stress reduction, different strategies may be required for different people and different circumstances.

The main objective in managing stress is to help the client to improve the quality of their lives and their resistance to stress by employing certain techniques, as well as making certain lifestyle changes. It is important to realise that as people react differently to stress, different techniques or combinations of techniques may be required for each individual.

Stress can only be eliminated if the root causes are recognised and resolved. However, there are ways in which the unpleasant effects of stress may be reduced.

Relaxation techniques

Physical relaxation is something which often appears easy but in reality is a skill that needs to be learned and practised.

By teaching clients physical relaxation techniques you can help them to take responsibility for their stress reactions and reduce the distress of many conditions.

Tensing muscles and holding breath when tense becomes habitual; the key to relaxation is training the body to feel tension and recognise when breathing reflects tension.

The body's reaction to stress involves breathing and muscle tension: the parts over which a person can gain control. The aim of relaxation is to control breathing and muscle tension in order to calm the mind and body.

Through learning physical relaxation, a person can learn to slow down their breathing, breathe deeply and relax their muscles. As the relaxation response starts to happen, other responses change automatically and as the breathing calms down and the muscles relax, the heart rate simultaneously slows down. With relaxation, the key is in gaining control over breathing and muscles: the rest will happen automatically as the body responds positively to being in a state of relaxation.

Relaxation can help to:

- maintain emotional and physical health
- aid restful sleep
- reduce the harmful effects of stress
- relieve muscular tension
- promote optimum oxygen levels for the body
- aid the body to recover and repair.

Breathing

Deep breathing is a very effective method of relaxation and works well combined with other relaxation techniques such as relaxation imagery, meditation and progressive muscular relaxation.

On inhaling, the intercostal muscles, abdominal muscles and the diaphragm contract in order to increase the volume of the thoracic cavity which causes air to pass into the lungs. While the breath is held, all these muscles remain tensed. When they relax, the volume of the thoracic cavity decreases as the muscles return to their original relaxed position. Comfortable, healthy breathing brings air down into the depth of the lungs and the body is able to relax as the breath is let out. When the body is still tense, breathing becomes fast and the muscles in the upper part of the chest take over to cause panting.

The experience of any physical or emotional stress will affect breathing. At times of stress, breathing becomes shallow and irregular, resulting in the brain being deprived of sufficient oxygen. This leads to a feeling of dizziness, inability to concentrate, and agitation. Learning how to breathe deeply helps to fill the body with positive energy and clears the mind. It can also help prevent a person from getting stressed, or can help them gain control more quickly when they are feeling stressed. Most people use only half of their lung capacity and breathe with their chest and not their diaphragm.

Below are two breathing exercises which may be taught to clients for self-help. It is important for clients to practise breathing exercises regularly, in order that they may be prepared to use them the next time they feel anxious and stressed.

Breathing exercises for successful stress control

Breathing exercise 1

Sit in a comfortable position and loosen tight clothing.

Place one hand on the chest and the other across the stomach.

Inhale deeply through the nose to fill the upper chest cavity and down to the lower part of the lungs, as if breathing into the stomach for a count of 6.

Exhale slowly to a count of 12, allowing the air to escape from the top of your lungs first before the lower part deflates.

Repeat this exercise 6–8 times.

Breathing exercise 2

Apply the first two fingers of the right hand to the side of the right nostril and press gently to close it. Breathe in slowly through the left nostril and hold for a count of 3.

Transfer the first two fingers to the left nostril to close it.

Breathe out slowly through the right nostril on a count of 3. Breathe in through the right nostril and hold for a count of 3 and while holding transfer the fingers to the right nostril and breathe out.

Repeat the exercise 6 times.

> ## *key note*
> After completing breathing exercises, clients should be advised to wait a few moments before getting up, in order to avoid dizziness.

Correct breathing is something which really needs to be practised often until it feels natural and it may then be utilised as a counterbalance to stress. Breathing properly enables the body to relax and regain its natural balance, whilst calming the mind. If a client has difficulty breathing correctly, it may be advisable for them to attend classes which involve structured breathing, such as yoga.

The effects of poor breathing on the body can be damaging in that it:

* weakens the nervous system

- encourages muscle tension
- starves the body of nutrients
- blocks the circulation
- weakens the immune system
- disturbs digestion.

Progressive muscular relaxation

This is a physical technique designed to relax the body when it is tense. It may be applied to any group of muscles in the body, depending on whether one area is tense or whether it is the whole body.

PMR is achieved by tensing a group of muscles so that they are as tightly contracted as possible. The muscles are then held in a state of tension for a few seconds and relaxed. This should result in a feeling of deep relaxation in the muscles.

For maximum effect, this exercise should be combined with breathing exercises and imagery (such as the image of stress leaving the body).

Relaxation exercise

Find a place where you can feel comfortable.

Close your eyes and pull your feet towards you as far as you can, hold them for a count of 5 and let them relax. Let them drop as if you are a puppet on a string and the string had broken.

Curl your toes as if you were holding a pencil, hold them for a count of 5 and then relax.

Tighten and tense the calf muscles, count to 5 and then relax.

Tighten and tense the thighs, press them tightly together, count to 5 and then relax, allowing them to fall apart.

Tighten the abdominal muscles, pulling in the muscles, count to 5 and then relax.

Tighten the muscles in the hips and the buttocks, count to 5 and then relax.

Arch the back and tense the back muscles, count to 5 and then relax.

Tense the shoulders by raising them to the ears, count to 5 and then drop them.

Lift your arms up with the hands outstretched as if you were reaching for something. Hold for a slow count of 5 and then let the arms drop down.

Tense the muscles in the forehead, count to 5 and then relax.

Tense the muscles around the eyes tightly, count to 5 and then relax.

Tense the muscles in the jaw and cheeks (as if gritting your teeth), hold for 5 and then relax.

By now you should feel relaxed and heavy, as if you are sinking into the floor or chair.

Check that all body parts are free from tension and if there are any areas left with tension, hold that part tense again before relaxing.

When you're ready, get up gradually, taking your time.

NB. This exercise will be easier to do if the instructions are on tape, preferably spoken by a person with a slow, calm and relaxing voice.

Imagery and visualisation

Imagery techniques can be useful to recreate a retreat from stress and pressure, by imagining a place or event that was happy and restful, and calling upon it to help manage a stressful period.

Imagery and visualisation are often more effective and real if combined with sounds, smell, taste and warmth. It is important to realise that visualisation is a very individual skill. Clients should be encouraged to call upon a happy experience, and that visualisation could be geared towards that image. Imagery and visualisation can often be enhanced by a relaxation tape which may be played while the client is receiving treatment and can be purchased for home use.

Meditation

This is a very effective way of relaxing as the idea is to focus your thoughts on relaxing for a period of time, leaving the mind and body to recover from the problems and worries that have caused the stress. Meditation can help to reduce stress by slowing down breathing, helping muscular relaxation, reducing blood pressure, and encouraging clear thinking by focusing and concentrating the mind. The key to meditation is to quieten the mind and focus completely on one thing.

With meditation, it is important for the body to be relaxed and in a comfortable position.

Meditation is a very personal experience and can involve a person sitting or lying quietly and focusing the mind, or it can be taught in a class situation.

Therapists may also facilitate meditation by using positive mental imagery and visualisation in order to help clients focus their mind on their imagery and lift themselves into a state of passive awareness in order to relax.

Relaxing at work

When a person spends hours sitting at a desk, driving or in meetings, tension can accumulate in the areas of the body most vulnerable to stress, such as the head, neck and shoulders.

Using a simple relaxation routine while at work can help to release tension, reduce stress and renew the body's energy to carry on working effectively.

Start by loosening any tight clothing (collar, tie, scarf) and removing your shoes.

5-minute stress reliever

Sit comfortably with your back supported against the back of the chair, your feet firmly on the ground and your hands and arms open and relaxed and supported by arm rests.

1 With a deep breath in, raise the shoulders towards the ears and hold them raised for a few seconds (be aware of the tension that may be accumulating in the shoulders); now take a long slow breath out and drop the shoulders down.
Repeat this exercise several times.

2 Now lift your right shoulder and slowly pop it backwards several times, ensuring that the arms are kept loose and relaxed. Repeat the exercise with the left shoulder. *Now pop both shoulders together. Repeat several times.*

3 Place your left hand on your right shoulder and squeeze gently and then release. Repeat the exercise down the right arm to the elbow. Repeat several times. Now place your right hand on your left shoulder and repeat the exercise.

4 Place your hands over your shoulders. As you exhale, let your head fall backwards and slowly draw your fingers over the clavicles (collar bones). Repeat several times.

5 Place your hands over the top of your head and gently pull your head gently downwards, feeling the slight stretch in the back of the neck. Hold this position for several seconds and then repeat.

6 Place the fingers of both hands at the base of your skull; apply slow circular pressures from the base of the skull and behind the ears, gradually working down the neck. Repeat several times.

7 Exhale and turn the head to the right side. Hold there for a few seconds and use the right hand to massage the right side of the neck from behind the eye down to the clavicle (collar bone). Repeat the exercise on the other side of the neck.

8 Now close your eyes and relax the muscles in your face. Be aware of your eye muscles, your jaw and your forehead. Place the fingers of both hands on each side of the temples and slowly massage in a circular motion, repeating several times.

9 Place the fingertips of both hands in the centre of the forehead and perform slow circular movements with both hands, working out towards the temples. Repeat several times.

10 Finish by cupping your hands over your eyes and holding for several seconds. This helps to release tension and tightness left in the face.

Clients can be encouraged to practise these exercises at least once a day during a break, and individual exercises may be used whenever they start to feel tense, to avoid stress building up.

Stress management is something which needs to be assessed in a holistic way, and will undoubtedly involve many other factors which include:

Welcoming change

It is important to realise that in implementing a stress management programme, there will be an element of change, and success will often depend on the adaptation to change. Changes in circumstances and lifestyle can be stressful; however, it is often the anticipation of the change that is more stressful than the change itself.

Attitude to stress

Attitude is a fundamental factor in stress management. A negative attitude can cause stress by alienating and irritating other people, whereas a positive attitude can help to draw the positive elements out of a situation and can make life more pleasurable and stress more manageable.

When the body is under stress, it is very easy to lose perspective; relatively minor problems can be perceived as threatening and intimidating. When faced with a seemingly overwhelming problem it may help to view the problem in a different way, for instance as a challenge or seeing what may be learned from it, whatever the outcome. It is important to be able to view mistakes as learning experiences, and realise that if something has been learned from an experience, then it has a positive value. Learning how to change the response to stress can help to transform it from a negative to a positive experience.

It may help to talk to someone who has had similar problems, or write the problem down in order to help put it into perspective. It is often helpful to break the problem down in order that it may be reduced to a smaller, more manageable size.

Positive thinking/cognitive therapy

Negative thoughts can cause stress as they can damage confidence and harm effective performance by stifling rational thoughts. Common negative thoughts are feelings of inadequacy, self-criticism, dwelling on past mistakes and worrying about how you appear to others.

Awareness of negative thoughts can be the first step to counterbalancing stress. It is important to write negative thoughts down and review them rationally, deciding whether they are based on reality. It is useful to counter negative thoughts with positive affirmations in order to change a negative thought into a positive one, such as 'I can do this'.

Stress from the environment

Disorganised living and working conditions can be a major source of stress. A well-organised and pleasant environment can usually make a large contribution to reducing stress and increasing productivity. Stress may be reduced in the environment by improving air quality, lighting, decoration, untidiness and noise levels. Natural light can lift moods and help prevent eyestrain. Creating order out of disorder can help clear a space mentally and physically to regain a state of calm.

When working in an office, it is advisable to consider the ergonomics of furniture as a potential source of stress. If you are working at a computer station, chairs should be checked for comfort and height and the keyboard and monitor comfortably positioned and at the right height. Taking a short break from computer/desk work every hour or so can help prevent tension and eyestrain from building up.

Health and Nutrition

Eating an unbalanced diet can cause stress to the body by depriving it of essential nutrients. Eating a well-balanced diet can help to eliminate chemical stress that may be caused by consumption of too much caffeine, too much alcohol, smoking, and food with high levels of sugar and salt.

Drinking more water may help to increase energy levels and the resistance to stress, by clearing the toxins from the bloodstream. Eating sensible well-balanced meals can help to calm or energise the mind and body and counteract the effects of stress.

The best defence against negative stress is a healthy and nutritious diet.

Implementing the following guidelines with diet and nutrition can help towards successful stress control:

- taking time out to eat properly (avoid working lunches)
- eat slowly and chew food well to aid digestion
- rest for a few minutes after eating
- eat fresh food to provide the body with essential vitamins and minerals
- avoid eating late at night to allow the body time to digest food properly
- avoid overeating, as it will decrease energy levels
- avoid eating if you are feeling angry, agitated or upset (practise relaxation techniques before eating).

A healthy diet to help beat stress will consist of:

- eating food rich in vitamins such as citrus fruits and dark green leafy vegetables
- eating foods rich in vitamin A and folic acid
- cutting back on alcohol, caffeine, refined sugars, salt and saturated fats
- eating iron-rich foods such as dried beans, peas and leafy green vegetables
- eating foods high in zinc and magnesium (seafood, whole grains and dried beans)
- eating balanced amounts of protein, fat, and carbohydrates to help provide the body with energy to be able to cope with stress
- eating plenty of whole, unprocessed foods (wholegrain bread and cereals, dried beans and peas, fresh fruit and vegetables, low-fat milk)
- drinking at least two pints of water a day.

Exercise

Taking frequent exercise is one way of reducing stress, as it helps to improve your health, relaxes tense muscles, relaxes the mind and helps induce sleep. Exercise can help to accelerate the flow of blood through the brain, helping the brain to function more clearly, and will remove waste products that have built up as a result of intensive mental energy. Exercise also releases chemicals called endorphins into the blood stream that give a feeling of wellbeing.

When considering incorporating exercise into a stress management programme, thought should be given to the type of exercise and its suitability to the individual, as if it is difficult or unenjoyable it may cause stress and may not be continued long enough to derive long-term benefits.

Taking time out

A successful way of reducing long-term stress is to take up a hobby where there is little or no pressure for performance. Long-term stress can also be reduced by taking time out for undirected activities such as reading a book, taking a walk, having a long bath, listening to music. It is important to take regular holidays or breaks in order to refresh mind and body and recharge energy levels. Taking a break can also help put problems into perspective.

Managing relationships (home and work)

Stress can be caused by relationships with other people and although it is not possible to change a person's personality, a change of attitude will often determine the amount of stress experienced from the situation.

A useful technique to employ when dealing with other people is to try to understand the way they think and why they feel the way they do. Unfortunately, it is human nature that people will often attempt to exploit a relationship at the expense of another person. In this case, it is important to project the right approach – by being positive, pleasant but assertive.

When dealing with a difficult, annoying or frustrating person, it is always a good policy to stay calm and neutral (take deep breaths) in order to be able to think more clearly and react more rationally. It is also important to be able to respect other people's opinions and to accept that some people or situations may not change.

Indian Head Massage as an antidote to stress

Holistic therapies such as Indian Head Massage can help clients to manage their stress as they provide a period of time away from everyday stresses in order to relax and regain a sense of physical and emotional balance. A combination of relaxation and holistic therapy programme can relieve tension and stress and allow the body energies to flow more freely. When the body reaches a state of relaxation tense muscles start to unknot, blood pressure starts to lower, breathing becomes more regular and deeper, and the mind drifts into a state of passive awareness.

Indian Head Massage is particularly effective as an antidote to stress as it relaxes and revitalises the mind and body, and can help with anxiety, tension and many stress-related conditions.

Other professional help

Although holistic therapies can provide a positive counterbalance to the negative effects of stress, it is important that a client does not become dependent on a therapist for any advice or service other than that which is associated with the chosen treatment.

Clients may need to consult another professional; for instance, if they are deeply depressed they may need to be referred to their GP or to a counsellor.

> *key note*
>
> It is unhealthy for a client to become reliant on a holistic therapist for their problems and see them as the one to provide a solution to their stress. The key to successful stress management is for clients to be able to recognise their own stress and for the therapist to help guide them as to how they may manage it.

NOTE:

Therapists should always take care to ensure that they remain objective with clients at all times and realise that by not taking responsibility for the client's problems they are in fact helping them to help themselves.

Time Management

By employing time management skills effectively, time can be utilised in the most productive and effective way. Time management can help to reduce stress by increasing productivity, therefore allowing more time to relax outside work activities.

The important factor in time management is to concentrate on results and not on activity, by:

- assessing the value of your time and how it may be used most effectively
- focusing on priorities, while deciding which tasks can be delegated and which may be dropped
- managing and avoiding distractions
- finishing work that has been started and working systematically
- learning when to say no and avoiding feeling guilty for doing so
- avoiding being someone else's time problem and reducing commitments
- having a planner for the weeks of the years, including a plan for holidays and leisure.

This can help to reduce the effects of long-term stress by helping to put things back into perspective, giving a feeling of control and direction and freeing more quality time to relax and enjoy life outside work.

Evaluating stress from experience

In a stress management programme, it is important to look back and re-assess in order to plan for the future. Planning ahead can help you to manage stress more effectively, rather than waiting for the distress signals. It is always useful to look back on a stressful situation in order to assess whether it was dealt with successfully and in order to decide what could be repeated or what needs to be changed.

Stress Management in the Workplace

Stress is a significant factor, costing billions of pounds a year, as it is thought that 60 per cent of absenteeism in the workplace is caused by stress-related disorders.

Over the last century, ever-increasing technological changes have led to a faster pace of life and to people being required to perform the job descriptions that may previously have been assigned to several people.

Stress occurs when the body is required to perform beyond its normal range of capabilities and the net results of this can be harmful to both individuals and organisations. It is also important to realise that stress can be a motivator and that people need a certain amount of pressure in order to stimulate them into action. Positive stress is the type of stress that gives the body a kick-start when needed. It is a known fact that people with too much time on their hands and not enough stimulus suffer from symptoms of stress, just as do those with too much work and too little time.

Companies are starting to realise that their staff members are more productive when they are able to deal with stress creatively and any factors that can help to reduce the damaging effects of stress can make the workforce happier and increase productivity.

Part of an action plan for stress management at work may include the following:

- learning to recognise the warning signals of stress and act on them to start taking control of stress responses
- enlisting the support of colleagues and not being afraid to talk about stressful situations in order to relieve some of the feeling of pressure
- taking regular breaks away from the desk or workspace and getting some fresh air (even if it means opening a window or door)
- paying attention to the ergonomics of office furniture and trying to keep your work-space uncluttered
- eating healthily and regularly
- eating slowly and digesting food properly
- learning to delegate and use time management skills – making a list and prioritising
- keeping a stress diary, noting the days when high stress levels are experienced and learning from these to help counterbalance the negative effects in the future
- setting realistic goals to avoid the stress of failing to meet an unrealistic deadline
- concentrating on one task at a time
- pause after completing one task before starting another
- planning activities for days off
- trying to view problems as challenges and as opportunities
- thinking positively – negative thought processes can be disabling and very destructive
- learning to see the funny side of stressful situations
- looking after yourself
- using relaxation techniques regularly.

Indian Head Massage as a counterbalance to stress in the workplace

Many companies and individuals are now aware of the costs negative stress can have on their company and their staff. Staff illness can lead to reduced productivity and increased pressure being placed on other individuals, leading to low morale and high staff turnover. Frequent complaints of work-related stress include the following:

'my neck and shoulders ache constantly from using the phone all day'

'I frequently suffer from headaches at work and feel under pressure all the time to meet tight deadlines'

'I never have time for a lunch hour as there is always too much work and not enough time to complete it in'

'I feel stressed-out and tired before I even start work and am too exhausted to enjoy a social life'

Comments like those above sound all too familiar to those suffering from the negative effects of stress at work, who could benefit from stress reduction techniques.

Some organisations have occupational health advisors who look after the welfare of their staff and are interested in ways in which staff stress levels may be managed effectively. Indian Head Massage is well suited to the work environment due to its portable nature. An area of the workplace (preferably private) can be assigned for the treatment, which is performed in an ordinary chair and is short enough in duration to be slotted into a break or lunch hour. It is also advantageous in that the client does not have to undress.

The benefits of Indian Head Massage to organisations and individuals are that it helps to:

- increase staff morale by alleviating depression and anxiety
- relieve stress and muscular tension
- relieve headaches, neck and back ache
- relieve eyestrain
- relieve mental and physical strain
- improve concentration levels, memory and mental alertness
- increase energy levels to improve productivity.

SELF-ASSESSMENT QUESTIONS

1 Which of the following statements is **false**?

   a stress is the imbalance between the demands of everyday life and the ability to cope

   b too much stress can affect a person's ability to function effectively

   c stress is caused by external pressures, such as work

   d stress can involve any interference that disturbs a person's emotional and physical well being.

2 Which of the following is **not** a symptom of long-term stress?

   a rapid breathing

   b digestive problems

   c excessive tiredness

   d mood changes.

3 Which hormone increases in production when the body is under stress?

   a thyroxine

   b adrenaline

   c oestrogen

   d oxytocin.

4 State three factors that may affect the body's capacity to deal with stress effectively.

5 Which of the following effects on the body are associated with the alarm stage of stress, as defined by Dr Hans Selye?

   a increased heart and ventilation rate

   b colds and flu

   c high blood pressure

   d anxiety and depression.

6 List six important components of an effective stress management programme.

Maintaining and Supporting Employment Standards

Competence in the workplace requires a therapist to support standards in the workplace in order to maintain employment. This role extends to supporting health, safety and security procedures when providing services to the general public and in safeguarding the safety of themselves, their colleagues and clients.

The success of a therapist lies not only in their ability to perform their own job roles effectively but to be able to contribute to the overall efficiency and operation of a business, upon which their livelihood ultimately depends.

By the end of this chapter, you will be able to understand and apply the following knowledge to your workplace practice:

chapter contents

- Workplace standards and industry codes of practice
- Hygienic precautions required for professional practice of Indian Head Massage
- Health, safety and security procedures in the workplace
- Professional codes of practice in the workplace
- Supporting and maintaining efficient workplace services and operations
- The implications of relevant legislation in relation to Indian Head Massage.

Workplace Standards and Industry Code of Practice

A therapist carrying out the professional practice of Indian Head Massage needs to understand that their work activities and responsibilities must comply with the rules of the individual establishment in which they are working.

Establishment rules lay down a benchmark of standards required by the workplace and are set according to the requirements of the individual business. They will include codes of professional dress, conduct and specific responsibilities.

Following is an example of establishment rules.

Establishment rules

It is each therapist's responsibility to ensure the following procedures and regulations are observed and adhered to during salon operational periods. These duties are required in line with establishment rules, health and safety policies, local bye-laws and awarding body guidelines.

Professional appearance

Workwear – all therapists must wear professional workwear for **ALL** practical sessions in the salon, in order to present a professional image of the establishment and to maintain hygiene.

Footwear – footwear should be low-heeled, comfortable, clean, enclosed at the toes and of smart and professional appearance.

Hair – should be clean, neatly styled and secured away from the face. It is important to tie long hair back, for hygienic and practical reasons.

Jewellery and accessories – hands and arms should be bare of jewellery, other than a wedding band. All other jewellery must be unobtrusive.

Hands – these should be kept as soft as possible and protected from harsh chemicals. Nails must be kept **short** and without **nail enamel**. Hands must be cleansed immediately before and after physical contact with the client.

Personal Hygiene – because of the close nature of therapy treatments, attention should be closely paid to maintaining personal hygiene to avoid offending a client with bad breath or body odour. Attention is also drawn to avoiding strong-smelling foods, smoking and the wearing of highly scented products when in close contact with clients.

Professional conduct

Reasonable and professional behaviour must be demonstrated by the therapist at all times, and workplace practices adhered to, including being punctual and fully ready for work, as required.

Therapists should adopt a professional attitude to clients, colleagues and staff at all times. This will include adherence to establishment rules and workplace policies, in order to promote a continuity of professional service within the workplace.

All therapists are to observe the salon's Code of Ethics at all times.

Health and safety

All therapists are reminded of the importance of health and safety and hygiene precautions and these must be observed at all times in accordance with the specific treatment/s provided.

Damages, breakages/accidents

All incidents, including damages, breakages or accidents, must be reported to the Salon Manager. All accidents to be recorded in the accident book.

Liaising with Colleagues

All therapists are to contribute to the efficiency of the salon operation by assisting fellow colleagues and informing them of any changes in procedures (client running late/client arriving early/client cancelled etc.).

Security

Windows and Doors

Please ensure that all windows and doors are secured at the end of each session.

Personal belongings

The salon is unable to accept liability for loss or damage to personal possessions while on the premises. Therapists must therefore be vigilant over their own property, as well as that of clients, and keep handbags and other items of value in a safe place.

Records

In order to maintain confidentiality, it is essential that client records and other confidential papers are secured and locked away when unattended.

In the event of any problems or breaches of security, these should be reported to the Salon Manager.

Dealing with clients

Greeting clients

Clients visiting the salon are to be attended to promptly and efficiently in a professional manner at all times. Therapists are responsible for greeting their own clients promptly at Reception, carrying out the treatment in a professional manner and booking the client's next appointment.

Processing client payments

It is each therapist's responsibility to ensure that the correct fee is taken for the treatment provided. This includes recording the treatment and payment made on the record of payments sheet, in order that a reconciliation may be made at the end of the session.

Record keeping

It is essential that a central record is kept of all salon treatments and that client confidentiality is observed at all times. It is each therapist's responsibility to ensure that all records are completed fully at the conclusion of the treatment and are updated accordingly.

Cost-effectiveness

It is each therapist's responsibility to ensure that cost-effective use of all resources is maintained. Because of the volume of products used in the clinic, please ensure that you split couch roll and use only a designated amount of products/towels etc. needed for each treatment, in order to avoid wastage.

NB. Attention is also drawn to carrying out treatments in a commercially acceptable time.

Maintaining of salon resources

All therapists are responsible for the preparation of their work area session prior to the client's arrival, and for tidying up and leaving the work area ready for re-use.

Equipment/resource cupboards

All items which are designated for storage in specific cupboards should be placed in the relevant cupboard on the shelf clearly marked for that item. The cupboard should always be kept clean and tidy, as should the items placed within.

Shortages of stock

All breakages, spillages, damages or shortages in salon stock are to be reported immediately to the Salon Manager for action.

Laundry

All dirty linen should be folded neatly into a dirty linen bag, ready for laundering.

Bins

All bins and waste must be emptied at the end of each session.

Final check
At the end of your working day, please ensure that:

- all waste has been removed and disposed of
- client records have been updated and filed away
- your work area is tidy and ready for re-use
- all electrical appliances have been switched off
- the salon has been left secure (windows locked, doors locked).

Maintaining a Hygienic Working Environment

A therapist is responsible for applying the appropriate hygiene procedures at all times, to:

- ensure compliance with legislative and workplace requirements
- prevent cross-infection and contamination
- promote client confidence.

Hygiene precautions

- A smart and hygienic appearance should be presented at all times (including attention to personal hygiene).
- All equipment should be disinfected regularly.
- Rubbish should be disposed of regularly, in a sealed bin.
- Open cuts or abrasions should be covered with a waterproof plaster.
- All jewellery should be removed from the client and the therapist (with the exception of wedding bands).
- All materials and consumables used should be clean and hygienic, ensuring that all container tops are secured tightly after use.
- Therapists' hands should be washed with an anti-bacterial soap/hand cleanser before and after each client.

Health and Safety

Health and safety procedures are of paramount importance in the workplace. The law demands that every place of employment is a healthy, and above all safe, place to work, not only for employees, but also for their clients and other visitors who may enter the workplace.

Failure to comply with legislation may have serious consequences, such as:

- claims from injured staff or clients
- loss of trade through bad publicity
- closure of the business.

Health and safety legislation

Health and Safety at Work Act 1974

The Health and Safety at Work Act provides a comprehensive legal framework to promote and encourage high standards of health and safety in the workplace. It covers a range of legislation relating to health and safety. Both the employer and employee have responsibilities under the Act.

The responsibilities of the employer

- Safeguard, as far as possible, the health, safety and welfare of themselves, their employees, contractors' employees and members of the public.

- Keep all equipment up to health and safety standards.
- Have safety equipment checked regularly.
- Ensure that the environment is free from toxic fumes.
- Ensure that all staff are aware of safety procedures, by providing safety information and training.
- Ensure safe systems of work.

The responsibilities of the employee

- Adhere to the workplace rules and regulations concerning safety.
- Follow safe working practices and attend training as required.
- Take reasonable care to avoid injury to themselves and others.
- Co-operate with others in all matters relating to health and safety.
- Not interfere or wilfully misuse anything provided to protect their health and safety.

The Health and Safety Executive (HSE) has produced a guide to the laws on health and safety and it is a requirement that an employer displays a copy of this poster in the workplace.

What health and safety law requires

The basis of British health and safety law is the **Health and Safety at Work Act 1974**. The Act sets out the general duties which employers have towards employees and members of the public, and employees have to themselves and to each other. These duties are qualified in the Act by the principle of 'so far as is reasonably practicable'. In other words, the degree of risk in a particular job or workplace needs to be balanced against the time, trouble, cost and physical difficulty of taking measures to avoid or reduce the risk. What the law requires here is what good management and common sense would lead employers to do anyway: that is, to look at what the risks are and take sensible measures to tackle them.

Management of Health and Safety at Work Regulations 1999 (the Management Regulations)

These generally make more explicit what employers are required to do to manage health and safety under the Health and Safety at Work Act 1974. Like the Act, they apply to every work activity.

The main requirement on employers is to carry out a **risk assessment**. Employers with five or more employees need to record the significant findings of the risk assessment. Risk assessment should be straightforward in a simple workplace such as a typical office. It should only be complicated if it deals with serious hazards, such as those on a nuclear power station, a chemical plant, a laboratory or an oil rig.

Besides carrying out a risk assessment, employers also need to:

- make arrangements for implementing the health and safety measures identified as necessary by the risk assessment
- appoint competent people (often themselves or company colleagues) to help them to implement the arrangements
- set up emergency procedures

- provide clear information and training to employees
- work together with other employers sharing the same workplace.

Other regulations require action in response to particular hazards, or in industries where hazards are particularly high.

If there are more than five employees, a written health and safety policy is required.

Besides the Health and Safety at Work Act itself, the following apply across the full range of workplaces:

1 **Management of Health and Safety at Work Regulations 1999**: require employers to carry out risk assessments, make arrangements to implement necessary measures, appoint competent people and arrange for appropriate information and training.

2 **Workplace (Health, Safety and Welfare) Regulations 1992**: cover a wide range of basic health, safety and welfare issues such as ventilation, heating, lighting, workstations, seating and welfare facilities.

3 **Health and Safety (Display Screen Equipment) Regulations 1992**: set out requirements for work with visual display units (VDUs).

4 **Personal Protective Equipment (PPE) Regulations 1992**: require employers to provide appropriate protective clothing and equipment for their employees.

5 **Provision and Use of Work Equipment Regulations 1998 (PUWER)**: require that equipment provided for use at work, including machinery, is safe.

6 **Manual Handling Operations Regulations 1992**: cover the moving of objects by hand or bodily force.

7 **Health and Safety (First Aid) Regulations 1981**: cover requirements for first aid.

8 **Health and Safety Information for Employees Regulations 1989**: require employers to display a poster telling employees what they need to know about health and safety.

9 **Employers' Liability (Compulsory Insurance) Regulations 1998**: require employers to take out insurance against accidents and ill health to their employees.

10 **Reporting of Injuries, Diseases and Dangerous Occurrences Regulations 1995 (RIDDOR)**: require employers to notify certain occupational injuries, diseases and dangerous events.

11 **Noise at Work Regulations 1989**: require employers to take action to protect employees from hearing damage.

12 **Electricity at Work Regulations 1989**: require people in control of electrical systems to ensure they are safe to use and maintained in a safe condition.

13 **Control of Substances Hazardous to Health Regulations 2002 (COSHH)**: require employers to assess the risks from hazardous substances and take appropriate precautions. In addition, specific regulations cover particular areas, for example asbestos and lead.

14 **Gas Safety (Installation and Use) Regulations 1998**: cover safe installation, maintenance and use of gas systems and appliances in domestic and commercial premises.

Management of Health and Safety at Work Regulations 1999

These are concerned primarily with:

- avoiding risks
- evaluating the risks which cannot be avoided
- combating the risks at source
- adapting the work to the individual, especially with regard to the design of workplaces, the choice of work equipment and the choice of working and production methods, with a view, in particular, to alleviating monotonous work and work at a predetermined work-rate and to reducing their effect on health
- adapting to technical progress
- replacing the dangerous with the non-dangerous or the less dangerous
- developing a coherent overall prevention policy which covers technology, organisation of work, working conditions, social relationships and the influence of factors relating to the working environment
- giving collective protective measures priority over individual protective measures
- giving appropriate instructions to employees.

Manual Handling Operations Regulations 1992

This legislation covers musculo-skeletal disorders primarily caused by manual handling and lifting, repetitive strain disorders and unsuitable posture causing back pain.

The regulations cover minimising risks from lifting and handling large or heavy objects and require certain measures to be taken such as correct lifting techniques to avoid musculo-skeletal disorders.

Cash handling

Under the Health and Safety at Work Act 1974, failure to provide a safe system of cash handling could lead to prosecution of the employer. Employers must therefore ensure compliance with this legislation and avoid sending an individual to the bank in a way that exposes the employee to risk.

Health and Safety (First Aid) Regulations 1981

Under these regulations workplaces must have first aid provision. The form it should take will depend on various factors including the nature and degree of hazards at work, what medical services are available and the number of employees.

The HSE booklet **COP 42 FIRST AID AT WORK (ISBN 0 11 885536 0)** contains an Approved Code of Practice and guidance notes to help employers meet their obligations. The number of first-aiders needed in the workplace depends primarily on the degree of hazards. If the workplace is considered to be low hazard (such as a holistic therapy clinic) there should be at least one first aider for every 50 employees. If there are fewer than 50 employees, there should always be an appointed person present when people are at work if no trained first-aider is available.

First-aiders must undertake training and obtain qualifications approved by the HSE. At present, first aid certificates are valid for three years. A refresher course should be started before a certificate expires, otherwise a full course will need to be taken.

First aid kits

First aid kits should contain only items that a first-aider has been trained to use. They should always be adequately stocked and should **not** contain medication of any kind.

A general purpose first aid kit will contain the following items: bandages, plasters, wound dressings, antiseptic cream, quick sling, eye pads, scissors, safety pins and vinyl gloves.

First-aiders should record all cases they treat. Each record should include at least the name of the patient, date, place, time and circumstances of the accident and details of the injury and treatment given.

Personal Protective Equipment at Work Regulations 1992

This legislation requires an employer to:

- provide suitable protective clothing and equipment for all employees to ensure safety in the workplace
- ensure that staff are adequately trained in the use of chemicals and equipment
- ensure that equipment is suitable for its purpose and is kept in a good state of repair.

Control of Substances Hazardous to Health Regulations 2002 (COSHH)

Regulations under this legislation require employers to regulate employees' exposure to hazardous substances which may cause ill health or injury in the workplace, and involves risk assessment.

Risk assessment involves making an itemised list of all the substances used in the workplace or sold to clients that may be hazardous to health. Attention is drawn to any substances which may cause irritation, cause allergic reactions, burn the skin, or give off fumes.

Instructions for handling and disposing of all hazardous substances must be made available to all staff and training provided, if required.

Manufacturers will usually supply information relating to their products, and therapists should be able to recognise hazard warning symbols on labels and packaging.

Gas Safety (Installation and Use) Regulations 1994

This legislation relates to the use and maintenance of gas appliances. All work carried out on gas appliances must be undertaken by installers who are registered under the CORGI scheme. The Rights of Entry Regulations 1996 gives Gas and HSE inspectors rights to enter premises and order the disconnection of dangerous appliances. (HSE inspectors will not normally be CORGI registered and cannot personally undertake any work on a gas appliance, including disconnection.)

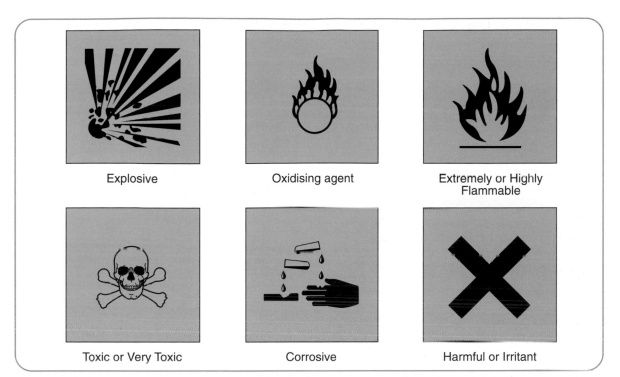

| Explosive | Oxidising agent | Extremely or Highly Flammable |
| Toxic or Very Toxic | Corrosive | Harmful or Irritant |

Hazard symbols

Electricity at Work Regulations 1989

Regulations under this legislation are concerned with safety in connection with the use of electricity.

It is recommended that electrical equipment be checked regularly (at least once a year) by a competent person such as a qualified electrician, in regard to correct fusing, no loose or frayed wires, insulation, earth leakage and so on.

All checks should be listed in a record book, stating the results of the tests and the recommendations and action taken in the case of defects. In the event of legal action, a record book may serve as important evidence.

Reporting of Injuries, Diseases and Dangerous Occurrences Regulations 1995 (RIDDOR)

This legislation requires that all accidents which occur in the workplace, however minor, **must** be entered into an accident register. This is a requirement of the Health and Safety at Work Act 1974.

An accident report form should contain the following information:

- details of the injured person (age, sex, occupation and contact details)
- date and time of the accident
- place where the accident occurred
- a brief description of the accident

- the nature of the injury
- the action taken
- signatures of all parties concerned (preferable).

The regulations under this legislation also require that if anyone is seriously injured or dies in connection with an accident in the workplace, or if anyone is off work for more than three days as a result of an accident at work, or if a specified occupational disease is certified by a doctor, then the employer must send a report to the local authority Environmental Health Department within seven days.

Local authority bye-laws

Larger local authority areas in the UK may impose their own legislation under which therapy establishments are licensed. Their position is not uniform and therefore practising therapists should obtain advice from the local Environmental Health Officer.

The Fire Precautions (Workplace) Regulations 1997

This legislation is for compliance with fire regulations and procedures in the workplace.

The Regulations require that:

- all premises have fire-fighting equipment that is in good working order
- the equipment is readily available and is suitable for all types of fire
- all staff are familiar with the establishment's evacuation procedures and the use of fire-fighting equipment
- fire escapes are kept free from obstruction and clearly signposted
- smoke alarms are fitted
- fire doors are fitted to help control the spread of fire.

It is a legal requirement for an employer to apply for a fire certificate if the business employs 20 or more staff.

It is important for all establishments to have set procedures in the event of a fire and that all staff are aware of it.

Fire-fighting and fire detection

Where necessary (whether because of the features of a workplace, the activity carried on there, any hazard present there or any other relevant circumstances) in order to safeguard the safety of employees in case of fire:

- a workplace shall, to the extent that is appropriate, be equipped with appropriate fire-fighting equipment and with fire detectors and alarms
- any non-automatic fire-fighting equipment shall be easily accessible, simple to use and indicated by signs
- an employer shall take measures for fire-fighting in the workplace, adapted to the nature of the activities and taking into account persons other than employees who may be present

- an employer shall nominate employees to implement those measures and ensure that the number of such employees, their training and the equipment available to them are adequate, taking into account the size of, and the specific hazards involved in, the workplace concerned
- an employer shall arrange any necessary contacts with external emergency services, particularly with regard to rescue work and fire-fighting.

Fire extinguishers

There are different fire extinguishers designed to deal with different types of fire.

From 1997, all fire extinguishers must be coloured red, but they all have different symbols and colour codes to show what type of fire they should be used for.

The main types of fire extinguishers are as follows:

Fire extinguisher colour	Contents	Type of fire
Red marking	Water	Paper, wood, fabrics and textiles (**not** on burning liquids, electrical or flammable metal fires)
Black marking	Carbon dioxide (CO_2)	Electrical fires, fats, grease, oils, paint, flammable liquids (**not** on flammable metal fires)
Blue marking	Dry powder	Electrical fires, oils, alcohols, solvents, paint, flammable liquids and gases (**not** on flammable metal fires)
Cream marking	Foam	Flammable liquids (**not** on electrical or flammable metal fires)
Green marking	Vaporising liquid	Electrical fires Flammable liquids (**not** on flammable metal fires)

These fire extinguishers are coded in order to allow quick and easy identification and to avoid using the wrong type and putting yourself and others in danger.

The main body colour of the extinguisher has changed over the past few years (any new extinguisher purchased or leased will be predominantly red). However, the type colour has remained the same.

NB. Any extinguishers that are not of the correct colour will be replaced when they become unserviceable.

Water extinguishers are usually colour-coded red.

Other types of extinguishers fall into different categories, namely:

- the entire body of the extinguisher is coloured in the type colour
- predominantly red with a 5 per cent second colour to indicate the contents of the extinguisher
- predominantly red with a boldly coloured block in the relevant colour, stating its type.

If you are in any doubt about the type of fire extinguisher to use in the workplace, it is advisable to contact your local Fire Safety Department for advice.

Emergency routes and exits

Where necessary in order to safeguard the safety of employees in case of fire, routes to emergency exits from a workplace and the exits themselves shall be kept clear at all times.

The following requirements must be complied with in respect of a workplace where necessary in order to safeguard the safety of employees in case of fire:

- emergency routes and exits shall lead as directly as possible to a place of safety
- in the event of danger, it must be possible for employees to evacuate the workplace quickly and as safely as possible
- the number, distribution and dimensions of emergency routes and exits shall be adequate, having regard to the use, equipment and dimensions of the workplace and the maximum number of persons who may be present there at any one time
- emergency doors shall open in the direction of escape
- sliding or revolving doors shall not be used for exits specifically intended as emergency exits
- emergency doors shall not be locked or fastened so that they cannot be easily and immediately opened by any person who may require to use them in an emergency
- emergency routes and exits must be indicated by signs
- emergency routes and exits requiring illumination shall be provided with emergency lighting of adequate intensity in the case of failure of their normal lighting.

Maintenance

The workplace and any equipment and devices shall be subject to a suitable system of maintenance and be maintained in an efficient state, in efficient working order and in good repair.

Environmental Protection Act 1990

This Act legislates for the improved control of pollution arising from certain industrial operations and other processes such as:

- waste on land
- the collection and disposal of waste
- offensive trades or businesses
- the extension of the Clean Air Acts to prescribed gases
- litter control
- radioactive substances
- genetically modified organisms
- potentially hazardous substances.

Special waste and non-controlled waste

If any kind of controlled waste is or may be so dangerous or difficult to treat, keep or dispose of that special provision is required, it is imperative to adhere to waste regulation authorities' rulings.

Waste other than controlled waste

A person who deposits any waste other than controlled waste, or knowingly causes or knowingly permits the deposit of any waste other than controlled waste, would be guilty of an offence and punished accordingly. This also applies if the waste is special waste and a waste management licence is not in force.

Dealing with spillages, breakages and waste in the workplace

When handling a **spillage**:

- wipe up immediately and warn staff and clientele. If the area is still wet, display a sign indicating the potential hazard.

When handling **breakages**:

- clear up immediately
- wrap up sharp items such as glass before placing them into the waste refuse.

When handling **waste**:

- dispose of in a covered bin
- remove daily.

Safety and security in the workplace

Therapists also require knowledge of security issues and measures in connection with premises, people and their belongings. Business requirements for the security of stock, equipment, money and records should be known.

The proprietor of a salon or clinic is required by law to ensure adequate security of their business premises.

The following steps may be taken to ensure maximum security. This is important not only for peace of mind but also for insurance requirements.

Security recommendations include:

* fitting locks and bolts on doors and windows
* installing a burglar alarm
* fitting security lights
* ensuring that there is a minimum number of key holders
* leaving a light on at night, preferably at the front of the premises
* ensuring that all windows and doors are checked before leaving the premises.

Money
* Have a safe for short-term storage of money and valuables.
* Always keep the till locked, with the minimum number of key holders.
* Never leave money in the till overnight.

Stock
A good stock control system is needed in the workplace in order to monitor the use of consumables and retail products, and this should be documented in a stock control book.

Recommendations for safeguarding stock include:

* always keeping supplies in a locked cupboard
* issuing keys to only a limited number of authorised staff
* have a locked cabinet for display purposes or use dummy stock to avoid shoplifting.

Records
In order to maintain confidentiality, it is essential that client records and other confidential papers are secured and locked away when unattended.

Personal belongings
It is not possible for therapists to take responsibility for a client's personal belongings when they attend for treatments. It is important for clients to be made aware of this by the salon displaying a disclaimer sign in a reception area.

When clients are removing jewellery, it is important for valuable items to be placed in a safe place for the duration of the treatment. In order to minimise risks, it is advisable to recommend that clients keep a minimum amount of money and valuables on them.

Staff should be vigilant over their own property as well as that of clients and keep handbags and other items of value in a safe place.

Health and Safety of the Client

Therapists need to have knowledge of health and safety in relation to the client, which includes risk assessment, contra-indications and contra-actions.

A therapist needs to understand fully that a contra-indication may mean a client being adversely affected by the treatment, or that treatment could be ineffective, and that an adapted or shortened treatment might be possible.

NB. Therapists must understand that diagnosis of a medical condition is the role of the medical profession, and therefore that suggestions should never be made to a client about a condition. It is the responsibility of the client to ask for medical advice concerning a contra-indication.

Any condition that does not appear to be normal should be brought to the attention of the client and medical consultation advised before treatment is given.

Contra-actions (adverse reactions) to treatment must be explained and avoided where possible. In the event of a contra-action, the corrective action to be taken and how to advise the client must be understood. It is also important to ensure that contra-actions are recorded.

Consumer Protection Act 1987

This Act provides the consumer with protection when buying goods or services to ensure that products are safe for use on the client during the treatment, or are safe to be sold as a retail product.

In the past, those injured had to prove a manufacturer negligent before they could successfully sue for damages. The Consumer Protection Act removed the need to prove negligence.

The Act provides the same rights to anyone injured by a defective product, whether the product was sold to them or not.

The Act also covers giving misleading price indications about goods, services or facilities. The term 'price indication' also includes price comparisons. To be misleading includes any wrongful indications about conditions attached to a price, about what you expect to happen to a price in the future and what you say in price comparisons.

It is essential to understand the implications of this legislation, including the promotion of special offers, as an offence could result in legal proceedings.

Sale and Supply of Goods Act 1994

As consumers of products and services, clients do have rights under this legislation which identifies the contract of sale that takes place between the retailer (the clinic/salon) and the consumer (the client).

This legislation amends the previous Act (Sale of Goods Act 1979), which was the first of the modern consumer laws and covers rights including the goods being accurately described without misleading the consumer.

The Sale and Supply of Goods Act 1994 is associated with the Supply of Goods and Services Act 1982, the Unfair Contract Terms Act 1977 and the Supply of Goods (Implied Terms) Act 1973.

These Acts cover consumer rights including goods being of satisfactory quality, the conditions under which goods may be returned after purchase and whether goods are fit for their intended purpose.

Trade Descriptions Act 1968 (amended 1988)

This Act prohibits the use of false descriptions or the sale of goods that have been described falsely. This Act covers advertisements such as oral descriptions or display cards and applies to quality and quantity as well as price and fitness for purpose.

It is important to understand this legislation, especially where the description is given by another person and repeated. To repeat a manufacturer's claim is to be equally liable for any false description contained in the claim.

Local Government (Miscellaneous Provisions) Act 1982

Part 8 of this Act provides local authorities with powers of registration of persons practising acupuncture, tattooing, electrical epilation and ear piercing, among other things. This applies to those operating from permanent premises or having home-visiting practices.

The primary concern of this legislation is within hygiene practices and may include qualifications. The precise bye-laws may vary between local authorities, as does the licence and inspection system involved. In areas where this is required, only those who are registered are allowed to practise both from permanent premises and by home visiting. Operators working under medical control (as in a hospital) are specifically excluded from registration.

Employers' Liability (Compulsory Insurance) Act 1969

This legislation requires the employer to take out and maintain an approved insurance policy with authorised insurers against liability for bodily injury or disease sustained by their employees in the course of their employment.

A certificate of employers' liability insurance must be displayed at each place of business for the information of the employees. Local authorities are specifically excluded from this Act.

Performing Rights Act (under Copyright, Designs and Patents Act 1988)

If a therapist is using relaxation music when carrying out treatments in the workplace it may be necessary to obtain a licence from Phonographic Performance Ltd (PPL) or the Performing Right Society (PRS). These are organisations that collect licence payments as royalties on behalf of performers and record companies, whose music is protected under the Copyright, Designs and Patents Act 1998.

Any use of music in treatment premises or waiting rooms, or music played on a switchboard holding system, is termed a public performance. The PPL and PRS have the backing of the Copyright, Designs and Patents Act 1988 and can take legal action against those who seek to avoid paying their licence fees.

However, it should be noted that a lot of music comes from composers who are not members of the above schemes. In such cases the music is 'copyright free' and no fee is due to PPL or PRS.

Therapists are advised to check the position with the supplier of the music.

Data Protection Act 1998

This legislation protects clients' personal information being stored on a computer. If client records are stored on computer, the establishment must be registered under this Act.

The Data Protection Act operates to ensure that the information stored is used only for the purposes for which it was given. Therefore none of the information may be given to any outsider without the client's permission.

Clients can seek compensation through the courts for any infringement of their rights established by giving information in the first instance for a specific purpose.

Businesses should therefore ensure that they:

- hold only information which is relevant
- allow individuals access to the information held on them
- prevent unauthorised access to the information.

Cosmetic Products (Safety) Regulations 2003

This legislation implements EEC regulations regarding the description of cosmetic products, their labelling, composition and marketing.

It is concerned with the supply of any cosmetic product which is liable to cause damage to human health when it is applied under:

a normal conditions of use; or

b conditions of use which are reasonably foreseeable, taking into account all the circumstances, including the cosmetic product's presentation, labelling, any instructions for its use and disposal and any other information or indication provided by the manufacturer, his agent or the person who supplies the cosmetic product on the first occasion that it is supplied in the Community.

Marking

Cosmetic products must be supplied in packaging which bears (in lettering which is visible, indelible and easily legible):

- a list of its cosmetic ingredients, (preceded by the word 'ingredients')
- the weight or volume
- the name or trade name of the product
- the address or registered office of the manufacturer of the product
- a 'Best Before' date (if the shelf life is less than 30 months)

- any particular precautions to be observed in use and any special precautionary information on a cosmetic product for professional use, in particular in hairdressing
- a means of identifying the batch in which the product was manufactured
- the function of the product, unless this is clear from its presentation.

Professional codes of practice

The role of a professional representative therapy body is in defining limitations on procedures and practices for public protection.

A professional therapist is bound by the rules of a professional representative therapy body (such as the Federation of Holistic Therapists) and its Code of Ethics, which exists to ensure that social, ethical and moral standards exist in a professional's day-to-day work.

Codes of ethics are rules of conduct binding on those who join a professional body. Infringement of these codes is taken very seriously by professional bodies and can result in penalties, including expulsion from membership.

A code of ethics also exists to determine the demarcation lines that enable a non-medical therapist to exist harmoniously in the industry with medical and medical-auxiliary practitioners. Therapists must, therefore, not practise beyond the scope of their profession.

Codes of ethics

Professional codes of ethics are standards of acceptable professional behaviour by which a person or business conducts their business.

Each professional association has its own code of ethics, to which it requires its members to adhere.

The following guidelines reflect, in general terms, a code of ethics expected from a professional therapist.

Therapists must:

- not treat any person who is suffering from a medical condition, and in the event of a client presenting a medical condition they should be referred to their GP
- conduct themselves in a professional manner and be courteous and respectful to a client at all times
- always bear in mind that their primary concern should be for the client and that they should practise their skills to the best of their ability at all times
- have respect for the religious, spiritual, social or political views of the client, irrespective of creed, race, colour or sex
- never abuse the relationship between themselves and a client
- act in a co-operative manner with other health care professionals and refer cases which are out of the sphere of the therapy field in which they practise
- explain the treatment and discuss any fees involved with the client before any treatment commences
- keep accurate, up-to-date records of treatments carried out on a client and the results, which should include the client's confidential details, a medical history, dates and details of treatment and any advice given

- never disclose client information without the prior written permission of the client, except when required to do so by law
- never claim to cure
- never diagnose a medical condition
- never give unqualified advice
- keep their personal and professional lives separate
- ensure that any advertising represents their business in the most professional manner
- ensure that their working premises comply with all current health, safety and hygiene legislation
- be adequately insured to practise the therapy in which they are qualified
- become a member of a professional association which sets high standards for the industry
- continue their own professional development.

Anti-discrimination practices

Anti-discrimination practices involve therapists ensuring equal treatment of all those with whom they come into contact.

It is each therapist's responsibility to examine their procedures and practices to ensure that they are non-discriminatory, and that cultural differences are fully respected when dealing with clients and colleagues.

A therapist needs to understand the nature and diversity of communities in that there are sub-groups of different economic, cultural or other divisions that co-exist within a geographical location.

Knowledge is therefore necessary of the existence of different communities within the larger community as a whole, in order to ensure that the provision of services encompasses the needs of the diversity of different groups within the local communities. This may involve communication with other professionals (medical and non-medical) within the community, to forge relationships that foster mutual respect and raise awareness to encourage integration of their chosen therapy within the community.

Therapists should understand that in the process of making professional contact with all parts of the community, they could improve knowledge and raise awareness of the benefits of the therapy to different groups within the area.

Anti-discrimination legislation

Discrimination occurs if an individual is treated less favourably than another on the grounds of race or sex.

Sex Discrimination Act 1975 (SDA) and Race Relations Act 1976 (RRA)

These provide that it is unlawful to discriminate on grounds of sex, marital status or race (defined as including colour, race, nationality or ethnic national origins). Both sex and race discrimination legislation specifically state that it is unlawful to discriminate against people in the following situations:

a recruitment (including job advertisements, interviews, refusal to offer employment)
b promotion
c transfer

d training
e benefits or facilities
f dismissal.

Protection for the Therapist and the Client

In professional practice, therapists may be in contact with various members of the community including the elderly, the infirm, those unable to give consent, special needs clients and clients of the opposite gender to the therapist.

Specific attention is drawn to the law regarding the protection of minors (persons below the legal age of consent). Therapists need to be aware that a minor should not be examined or treated unless a parent or guardian is present, or has given written permission for examination and a chaperone is present.

Specific precautions also exist in relation to those individuals in specific categories (the elderly, the infirm, those unable to give consent, special needs clients). In the treatments of these client groups, attention is drawn to the need for a companion, or appropriate adult (such as a carer), to be present to offer protection for the individual and the therapist. Any special precaution should be considered and requested before any treatment is undertaken.

A competent therapist needs to be sensitive to apparent signs of abuse, which could be in the form of physical, verbal, mental (bullying or discrimination), sexual, neglect or self-harming. However, it is imperative that under no circumstances must the therapist make comments or judgements, as this is outside their professional sphere.

Therapists must understand that their role is in adopting a supportive but professional attitude at all times, but at no time should they become directly involved.

Therapists need to be aware that the client may exhibit non-verbal signs indicating anxiety or concern and these should be observed and responded to appropriately.

Any signs of prior abuse should be noted by the therapist and treated confidentially within the law. Therapists need to be aware of any signs of inappropriate behaviour (which may include an action or statement from a minor not appropriate to their age, signs of being bullied, withdrawn or introverted behaviour, or may be in the form of bullying and discrimination). Therapists have a duty to report any abnormal statement, event or observation to a senior person in the establishment, and request advice if in any doubt as to how to proceed.

Providing a safe working environment

Therapists need to be aware of special precautions to ensure that clients do not feel vulnerable or at risk at any time.

The working environment in which the therapist practises must allow clients to feel comfortable and at ease at all times. Treatment processes should be not be invasive and all procedures must be explained to the client beforehand to ensure their consent is given for treatment to proceed.

Special precautions that therapists need to be aware of include having someone else nearby, working in an easily accessible working area and checking clients' details before offering treatment. As far as therapists are concerned, for personal protection they may refuse to treat anyone they have concerns about.

A therapist must exhibit professional conduct at all times, to allay fears of any inappropriate behaviour. In addition, therapists may themselves be subject to unwanted attention and therefore must know how to avoid giving misleading signals.

Legislation for the protection of minors

Children Act 1989
The Children Act of 1989 came into effect in 1991. It is an important piece of legislation concerning children and the way they are treated.

The Children Act gives children rights in that they should be consulted, listened to, protected and given their chance to voice their feelings and opinions. Most importantly, the Act has given children a voice in that it recognises that they should be treated with respect, and as individuals.

The key points of the Children Act are as follows:

* children's welfare in both private and public sectors is made a priority
* recognition that children are best brought up within their families, wherever possible
* aims to prevent unwarranted interference in family life
* requires local authorities to provide services for children and families in need
* promotes partnership between children, parents and local authorities
* improves the way that courts deal with children and families
* gives right of appeal against court decisions
* protects the rights of parents with children being looked after by local authorities
* aims to ensure that children looked after by local authorities are provided with a good standard of care.

Protection of Children Act 1999
This Act requires a list to be kept of persons considered unsuitable to work with children. It also makes provisions to extend the power of the regulations of the Education Reform Act 1988. It is also designed to enable the protection afforded to children to be extended to persons suffering from mental impairment.

NB. The Criminal Records Bureau may be consulted by employers of people with access to minors.

Youth Justice and Criminal Evidence Act 1999
This Act makes provision for the referral of offenders under 18 to youth offender panels. It includes the giving of evidence or information for the purposes of criminal proceedings and makes pre-consolidation amendments relating to youth justice.

Crime and Disorder Act 1998

This Act includes provisions for preventing crime and disorder, including certain racially-aggravated offences. It also includes abolishment of the death penalty for treason and piracy. It makes further provision for dealing with offenders and with respect to remands and committals for trial and the release and recall of prisoners.

Sex Offenders Act 1997

This Act primarily requires persons who have committed certain sexual offences to notify the police and to provide information in relation to the offences.
Any person convicted of a sexual crime will be placed on the Sex Offenders Register.

Care Standards Act 2000

This Act establishes a National Care Standards Commission. It covers the registration and regulation of children's homes, independent hospitals, independent clinics, care homes, residential family centres, independent medical agencies, domiciliary care agencies, fostering agencies, nurses agencies and voluntary adoption agencies. The Act also covers the regulation and inspection of local authority fostering and adoption services. It establishes a General Social Care Council and a Care Council for Wales and covers the registration, regulation and training of social care workers. Within the UK it establishes a Children's Commissioner for Wales in order to make provision for the registration, regulation and training of those providing child minding or daycare. It also makes provision for the protection of children and vulnerable adults and covers the law about children looked after in schools and colleges.

Children (Leaving Care) Act 2000

This Act covers provisions for children and young persons who are being, or have been, looked after by a local authority.

Human Rights Act 1998

This Act is to give effect to the rights and freedoms guaranteed under the European Convention on Human Rights (ECHR).

Author's Note

Whilst the Acts and Regulations mentioned in this book are current at the time of writing, legislation is constantly changing and being amended regularly. Good sources of information on the most current legislation and amendments can be found at *http://www.legislation.hmso.gov.uk/acts.htm* and *http://www.ukonline.gov.uk*

Maintaining Operations and Services

The role of a therapist in the context of the workplace is not merely in the provision of treatments, but in monitoring and maintaining the operations to meet the requirements of both the establishment and the client. They are concerned with matters that help to make a business run smoothly and efficiently, with the ultimate aim of clients who are satisfied with the service provided, and the result of repeat business.

Therapists are expected to understand what is required to support workplace efficiency, within their given area of responsibility.

There are several important factors to take account of when working as a therapist, in order to monitor and maintain the standard of service offered to clients.

It is important not only to be able to perform a skill competently but to be able to apply it in a way which is commercially acceptable.

In the workplace, therapists have a responsibility to their manager or supervisor, to their clients and to their colleagues.

Responsibilities of a therapist to a supervisor

These are to ensure that they:

- adhere to the establishment's rules
- understand and adhere to legislation in relation to the provision of services
- report any hazard or potential danger observed in the workplace
- have a sincere commitment to provide a high standard of work, to enhance the reputation and image of the establishment
- carry out work practices with honesty and integrity
- complete records fully and accurately
- work within own initiative to make best use of time at work
- provide a high standard of work to ensure client satisfaction and repeat business
- create a good working relationship with other colleagues to enhance a good working environment
- avoid wastage of resources
- make recommendations for improvement in workplace practices, where appropriate
- understand how their job role contributes to the success of the business.

Responsibilities of a therapist to a client

These are to:

- treat clients with dignity and respect
- respond to clients' requests politely and efficiently
- accurately inform them of the services provided by the establishment
- provide treatment only when there is a reasonable expectation that it will be advantageous to the client
- take appropriate measures to protect the client's right to privacy and confidentiality
- provide a high standard of service to ensure client satisfaction and the fostering of repeat business
- make recommendations for future treatments that would benefit the client
- make recommendations for home care products that may enhance the client's condition.

Responsibilities of a therapist to their colleagues

These are to:

- create a good working environment by being friendly, helpful and approachable
- share responsibilities fairly to enhance a good team spirit
- ensure good communication channels to enable them to pass on messages promptly and record messages accurately
- inform others of any changes in establishment procedure.

Maintaining effective relationships with colleagues

A successful business depends on a good image and reputation, but also depends on the way in which staff work together as a team to maintain the image and professionalism of the establishment.

Working with colleagues as a team helps enhance smooth operations and promotes a pleasant working environment and a friendly atmosphere.

Working as a team involves:

- building a good rapport with each other
- understanding each other's responsibilities
- working efficiently within your own job responsibilities
- responding to each other's requests politely and co-operatively
- providing support and assistance when required
- working together for the needs of the business.

Communication is essential when working with others in a team; regular meetings can help to maintain effective working relationships.

Meetings provide an opportunity to:

- identify and resolve problems in the workplace
- avoid breakdown in communication and misunderstandings
- contribute and exchange ideas on how workplace practices may be enhanced
- identify training needs
- maintain good working relationships.

Communication skills

Whether a business is small or large, its success relies on good communication to promote good understanding and efficient working relationships. Communication skills are extremely important when there are several colleagues working together. If communication breaks down, it can have a dramatic effect on the service given and the overall efficiency and image of the establishment.

It is therefore important for a therapist to be able to communicate effectively with clients, colleagues and other visitors who may visit or telephone the establishment.

Communication skills may be used to:

- identify clients' needs
- inform clients about a service
- inform clients and colleagues of changes in procedures and problems arising
- maintain workplace records
- pass on recommendations for improving employment standards.

Communication skills involve verbal communication, listening, non-verbal communication and written communication.

- **Verbal communication** – this involves sending and receiving information and is a co-operative effort between two parties. In order to facilitate effective verbal communication it is important to pause periodically in order to verify that the message received was the message intended. In this way, alternations and corrections to the conversation may be made.
  The objective of verbal communication is to be heard and understood.
  For clarity, it is important to choose words which convey intent clearly, concisely and tactfully.

- **Listening** – although it is important to facilitate effective verbal communication, it is equally important to have good listening skills in order to develop optimal client–therapist/client–colleague relationships. Effective listening involves understanding and evaluating the person's needs, including the tone and emotion in which the message is delivered. The objective of listening is focusing on understanding the message heard.
  Good communication may be enhanced by maintaining eye contact, nodding, using verbal phrases or facial expression in order to encourage the speaker to continue.
  When listening it is important for therapists to clarify information received from clients or colleagues in order to ensure that they understood the message correctly.

- **Non-verbal communication** – this involves messages transmitted other than by the spoken word and may be exhibited by posture, gestures and facial expressions.
  Non-verbal communication often projects more information about how a person is feeling and their emotions.
  As a therapist's role is in dealing with people, it is helpful to be aware of body language as this may have more meaning than the spoken word.

- **Written communication** – an efficient working environment providing services to clients relies on accurate, legible record keeping, which is kept up to date.
  Records may be either computer-based or handwritten.
  Written communication may involve the recording of messages to colleagues to ensure continuity of service, or the completion of client records in the workplace to ensure therapeutic continuity.
  In the workplace, it is very important that all messages are recorded accurately to ensure continuity of operation and services.
  Written communication should be clear, dated and timed, along with the action required. It should also be placed in a place where the person it is intended for will notice it.

Client records should be completed fully, accurately and legibly at the time of the treatment and stored securely and confidentially.

Responding to clients' requests

As clients are at the centre of every business it is essential for therapists to respond to their requests promptly, accurately and enthusiastically.

Requests for information may come from a telephone enquiry, a personal call to the workplace or a written request.

It is important to assume a friendly and approachable manner when dealing with clients' requests and to use phrases such as 'How may I help you?'.

It is also important to provide accurate information on treatments, such as:

*   the benefits of the services
*   the cost (of individual and courses of treatment)
*   the treatment duration
*   any pre-treatment advice
*   how often the client should attend, for maximum benefit.

Providing as much useful information as possible at the time of request will increase the chances of the client booking an appointment and, even if the client does not book immediately, it will certainly give them a good impression of the professionalism of the establishment.

The best source of information should be the professional themselves (the therapist). However, when this is not possible, it is important to consider that leaflets and brochures may also help to sell treatments to clients. The information contained within leaflets and brochures should therefore be educational and informative to increase client awareness of the treatment as well as being attractive enough to stimulate interest.

Quality Assurance

Every business, however small, should have a quality assurance policy in order to ensure that its services and operation are conducted in a systematic way.

Quality assurance policies help to monitor the quality and standard of the service provided and are useful in analysing whether the client's needs are met efficiently, effectively and consistently.

Effective ways of monitoring quality assurance include:

*   examining your own workplace practice and how it relates to client needs and the needs of the business
*   ensuring that you don't become complacent and that you continue updating your skills and knowledge
*   distributing client satisfaction questionnaires

- introducing a client suggestions box
- implementing changes based on recommendations from clients and staff.

Encouraging communication with clients on a regular basis can help to monitor the quality assurance policy of the establishment.

Cost-effectiveness

Efficient work practice requires a therapist to perform a skill to the required standard of the establishment and the industry, and in a time which is considered to be commercially acceptable.

Cost-effectiveness in terms of the workplace means maintaining treatment times and minimising waste in order to avoid loss of revenue for the establishment.

Therapists need to be aware that by adhering to their appointment times and avoiding wastage they are in fact helping to preserve the business's precious resources and thereby helping to maintain their security of employment.

SELF-ASSESSMENT QUESTIONS

1   The legislation that exists to require employers to carry out risk assessment in the workplace is

   a   Management of Health and Safety at Work Regulations 1999

   b   Workplace (Health, Safety and Welfare) Regulations 1992

   c   Personal Protective Equipment Regulations 1992 (PPE)

   d   Health and Safety (Display Screen Equipment) Regulations 1992.

2   A written health and safety policy is required when there are

   a   10 or more employees

   b   5 or more employees

   c   3 or more employees

   d   20 or more employees.

3   How many first-aiders are required to every 50 employees in a low-hazard workplace?

   a   at least 3

   b   at least 5

   c   at least 1

   d   at least 2.

SELF-ASSESSMENT QUESTIONS

4 Which of the following items should **not** be enclosed within a first aid kit?

   a wound dressings

   b plasters

   c medication

   d disposable gloves.

5 Which legislative Act exists to regulate an employee's exposure to hazardous substances?

   a Personal Protective Equipment at Work Regulations 1992

   b Control of Substances Hazardous to Health 1998 (COSHH)

   c Reporting of Injuries, Diseases and Dangerous Occurrences Regulations 1995 (RIDDOR)

   d Noise at Work Regulations 1989.

6 If client records are stored on a computer, the establishment must be registered under

   a Performing Rights Act

   b Trade Descriptions Act

   c Data Protection Act

   d Consumer Protection Act.

7 By law, what insurance certificate must be displayed in a place of work?

   a public liability

   b employers' liability

   c professional indemnity

   d personal injury indemnity.

8 It is a legal requirement for an employer to apply for a fire certificate if a business employs

   a 30 or more staff

   b 50 or more staff

   c 20 or more staff

   d 10 or more staff.

SELF-ASSESSMENT QUESTIONS

9 What legislation requires a list to be kept of persons considered unsuitable to work with children?

   a   Children Act 1989

   b   Protection of Children Act 1999

   c   Sex Offenders Act 1997

   d   Crime and Disorder Act 1998.

10 The hazard symbol that shows a skull and crossbones is used to indicate items which are

   a   highly flammable

   b   corrosive

   c   explosive

   d   toxic.

11 Which colour extinguisher should **not** be used to extinguish an electrical fire?

   a   black

   b   blue

   c   cream

   d   green.

12 Which of the following fire extinguishers should **not** be used on a fire caused by flammable liquids?

   a   black

   b   red

   c   cream

   d   blue.

Promotion and Marketing

9

Marketing is the means by which you tell potential clients what you have to offer and how it will benefit them.

In order to be successful in business, it is not enough for therapists to have excellent skills in the therapy they practise; they also need to get to grips with the important skill of marketing. Holistic therapists need to consider the marketing of services such as Indian Head Massage carefully as they are not looking to sell large volumes of consumer goods; it is a specialist market and the marketing must therefore be selective.

By the end of this chapter, you will be able to:

chapter contents

- Understand the fundamental issues of marketing and promotion
- Design a marketing plan for business success in Indian Head Massage.

Marketing in the holistic therapy industry is educational and is about raising awareness of who you are and what you do. It is important for therapists to consider that marketing is about matching service to clients' needs and therefore the focus is not so much on selling but on identifying needs. The key to successful marketing is to view every aspect of your marketing through the client's eyes and match their needs and desires to your products and services.

Marketing involves finding out:

- who your potential clients are
- what their needs are
- how much they would be prepared to pay for the service
- where they are and how to reach them
- how often they would visit.

Researching Clients

It is essential to use market research to assess the needs of the market. Knowing and understanding who your potential clients are is crucial to devising a marketing plan and deciding whom to target in advertising and promotion.

Market research enables you to identify potential clients, discover what influences them and find out how to reach them. Knowing the market then enables you to refine the message you wish to send to potential clients. There are very few services that will appeal to everyone; there is always a sector of the market that is going to be more inclined to buy. Therefore you need to find out who this sector is and focus the attention of your marketing on them.

When building client profiles, it is helpful to consider the following factors:

- age
- gender
- income
- interests
- location.

Gathering Client Information

As clients are at the centre of every business, it is vital to find out about them and what they want. Carrying out marketing surveys using questionnaires is an effective way of gathering information. A great deal of thought needs to be given to the design of a marketing questionnaire in order to give both quantitative and qualitative results.

When designing marketing questionnaires, it is important to keep questions short, simple and to the point in order to get an exact answer. If questions are structured it is simpler and quicker for the respondent to reply. Another important consideration is the type of questions to ask. Closed questions require only yes/no/don't know responses, while open questions are such that the respondent has to answer in their own way.

When designing questionnaires it is also important to remember to avoid pre-judging the participant's response: in other words, not assuming that you know what they are going to say. Neither should you leave them with no alternative but to agree with you.

In order to get the best results from your marketing questionnaire, bear in mind the following:

- keep it simple, attractive, interesting and relevant
- include a short introduction to the questionnaire in order to stimulate the respondent's enthusiasm and motivation to complete it
- offer an incentive to complete the questionnaire (such as a free prize or entry into a free prize draw)
- make it known to the respondents that there is a deadline for reply to the questionnaire.

You may wish to carry out a pilot survey on a group of individuals (friends, family, colleagues); however, check that the individuals concerned are among the right category of a potential client, otherwise this may prove to be a fruitless exercise.

Following is an example of a market research questionnaire for Indian Head Massage.

Indian Head Massage Questionnaire

Indian Head Massage is a traditional massage treatment originating from India. It involves the application of massage technique to the upper back and shoulders, upper arms, neck, face and scalp. The treatment is applied through the clothes, with the recipient remaining seated in a chair.

Indian Head Massage has many benefits, including helping to relieve muscular tension, relieving headaches and reducing stress levels.

This questionnaire is designed to establish current levels of awareness and interest in Indian Head Massage.

1   Have you heard of Indian Head Massage before?   **Yes/No**

2   If yes, when did you hear about it?

_____

_____

3   Do you experience any of the following on a regular basis?

high stress levels? ☐   muscular tension in the back, neck or shoulders? ☐

headaches? ☐   eyestrain? ☐   anxiety? ☐   depression? ☐

poor concentration levels? ☐

4   What measures do you take (if any) to help with any of the above?

_____

_____

5   Would you be interested in trying a treatment?   Yes/No

6   Would you like further information on Indian Head Massage and its benefits?   **Yes/No**

Thank you for your time and co-operation in completing this form. If you would like further information or would like to book a complimentary introductory treatment, please give your details below.

Name _____

Address _____

Telephone Number   Work: _____   Home: _____

Client surveys are useful tools in market research in that by gaining the client's input they:

- demonstrate your desire to offer the best possible service
- help you to fulfil the client's needs
- direct you towards potential sales triggers
- guide you towards potential strengths and weaknesses.

If sending out market research questionnaires, always make the response easy for the client by providing a stamped addressed envelope.

As Indian Head Massage involves a personal and specialised service, it tends to appeal to certain segments of the market. By selecting a target market it enables you to modify your advertising and promotional activities to appeal to a specific group.

Consider the type of clientele you want to attract or, if you have an existing clientele, examine who is already using your services and what they have in common.

When targeting client markets it is wise to have more than one sector, the number being dependent on your preference, expertise and the size of your practice.

In order to make marketing more effective, it is helpful to create a niche market by addressing the needs of a specific group of people. Your name then becomes linked with providing a particular service for a particular target group.

Assessing Marketing Needs

Marketing needs will be dependent on the following factors:

- your target market
- the size of your practice
- the amount of money you can afford
- the amount of time you can devote.

If you are a therapist starting out in business and do not have a large clientele, more time and energy can be devoted to making contacts and giving talks and presentations to help get your name and what you do known. The activities involving client education and awareness will be low-cost but time-consuming.

If you are an established business, you may have the financial budget to concentrate on other marketing methods such as targeted advertising or mailshots to announce the introduction of a new service such as Indian Head Massage into the business. An important factor to consider in marketing is that it takes time and money to become known in business.

Compiling a marketing plan

Once you have established where the market for Indian Head Massage is and how extensive it is, the next stage is to put all the findings together in the form of objectives – this will form a marketing plan. A marketing plan will form the basis of how you intend to promote the service to generate clients. Before compiling a marketing plan, it is essential to carry out a **SWOT** analysis in order to self-assess your Strengths, Weaknesses, Opportunities and Threats in order to be realistic in your plan.

STRENGTHS – these may include:

- specialism
- location of the business
- pricing
- the opening hours
- personality
- customer service
- flexibility.

> *key note*
>
> A marketing plan should also include your Unique Selling Point (USP) which is what makes your business and service different.

WEAKNESSES – possible weaknesses may be:

- lack of experience
- opening hours
- location
- range of skills offered.

OPPORTUNITIES – these could include:

- expansion into other sectors of the market, e.g. the workplace.

THREATS – potential threats may include:

- local competition.

Getting the balance right in marketing

Successful marketing usually involves a mix of different methods and the chemistry or 'mix' has to be right for the individual business.

Marketing can be divided into four factors and each of these will influence how you develop your marketing plan. Marketing can be seen as a balancing act and if adjustments are made to one or more of the four factors, then a compensating adjustment has to be made among the other factors in order for the approach to be balanced.

PRODUCT/SERVICE – this includes the features and benefits of the product/service being offered, including the quality of service. For marketing to be effective, it is important to create a demand.

With products and services, it is also important to consider the image of the business being projected by the service itself, the marketing material and the staff.

PRICE – this is the cost of the service to the client. When setting prices for services it is vital to consider the following:

- charge enough to cover your overheads and enough to meet your expenses and make a profit
- charge what clients are prepared to pay
- be in line with your competitors.

PLACE – this is where you are located in relation to your clients. Careful consideration needs to be given to the location and opening hours of the business to ensure that the service is available to potential clients.

Location is an important factor in business; it affects the distribution of services.

Because of the portable nature of Indian Head Massage, therapists should consider the many locations or settings in which the therapy may be practised (e.g. in the workplace, in hairdressing salons and hospitals as well as beauty spas and clinics).

PROMOTION – the objective of promotion is to become known and to create a desire in potential clients to use your services.

The promotion of services such as Indian Head Massage is largely educational in nature and is the means by which potential clients learn who you are, what you do and how your services will benefit them.

In the holistic therapy industry it is important for therapists to realise that they are marketing themselves as well as their treatments.

Marketing is the art of promoting yourself and the services you offer in order to attract clients.

There are many marketing strategies that can be used to sell the services you intend to offer. However, one of the most important attributes for a holistic therapist is to have self-confidence, a positive attitude and belief in themselves and their abilities.

As the holistic therapy business is a personal service, it is essential that therapists feel confident enough to sell their services and products to potential clients.

In order to be able to sell a service or product effectively, it is important for a therapist to:

- know the services well enough and have enough experience to be able to sell their benefits to potential clients
- be aware of the services of competitors and have identified their strengths and weaknesses
- be able to sell solutions
- identify with the potential client's needs and personalise the sale.

Personality selling

The concept of personality selling is very important in business. Some clients may decide whether to have a treatment based on factual information. In this case the benefits of the treatment need to be stressed in a very factual and analytical way.

Other clients may need to have a picture created for them, enhanced by imaginative therapeutic words to stimulate their interest.

> ### *key note*
> Some therapists may feel uncomfortable with the idea of selling and may need to attend sales training in order to enhance this very important skill.

No amount of advertising can make up for the personal touch and with Indian Head Massage it is best to consider the direct and more personal approach first and turn personal skills to your advantage. By creating a positive environment for treatment provision, therapists can sell through one of the most powerful senses – the therapeutic touch. When planning advertising and promotion, it is essential to use a mix of methods in order to reach different target markets and to help evaluate the overall effectiveness of the activities.

The direct approach to marketing and promotion

Personal recommendation/word of mouth

This is the most valuable form of advertising for personal treatments like Indian Head Massage. Once a therapist has established a reputation for excellent customer service and quality skills, a satisifed client will automatically recommend the service to another potential client. It is important for therapists to tell as many people as possible about Indian Head Massage and communicate their enthusiasm. Positive enthusiasm is infectious and even if the person you are speaking to does not need the information, they may pass it on to someone who does. The power of the spoken word is very effective in the marketing of services.

Talks and demonstrations

Talks and demonstrations are an effective way of presenting the service to a targeted group and they usually work best when presented together.

Talks should be informative and educational in nature (they should tell potential clients how Indian Head Massage will benefit them) and the demonstration should show the target audience the effects and help to break down barriers or pre-conceptions they may hold about the therapy.

It is useful to identify the needs of the target audience prior to the presentation, as this gives the therapist the advantage of being able to personalise the session.

Talks and demonstrations are best limited to a maximum of 30–40 minutes, with time left to answer questions and to distribute business cards and literature.

The focus of the talk should be about identifying with and providing solutions to the client's needs.

A useful checklist when preparing for talks is to:

- find out as much as possible about the target group before the talk
- confirm the number of people that will be attending
- check out the venue and its suitability
- plan out the talk with a basic outline format
- have a plentiful supply of literature to hand out
- prepare a list of possible questions you may be asked
- take some relaxation music to help create a relaxing ambience
- aim to involve the audience in the session (encourage questions or volunteers on whom to demonstrate)
- take your appointment book with you!

Exhibitions

Exhibitions are an effective way to communicate with lots of potential clients in one place. They are a useful way of distributing brochures and leaflets and to persuade new clients to watch a demonstration of a new service and sample it. When exhibiting at a show it is important to ensure that it is the right type of show for the image of the business and to speak to people who have attended the show in order to gain feedback from them.

In order to project the right image at an exhibition it is important to ensure that:

- the stand looks attractive, neat and tidy
- the stand is accessible and situated to your best advantage
- staff manning the stand look warm and welcoming, and are approachable to talk to
- there is space for people to browse without feeling intimidated.

It is also important, if possible, to take the names and contact numbers of those who visited the stand in order that you may contact them after the exhibition.

Building a referral network

This is one of the most successful and inexpensive ways of creating new business.

Current satisfied clients are one of the most effective means of advertising.

Referrals can be encouraged by:

• offering existing clients incentives to introduce new clients to use your service
• establishing links with other professionals by making yourself and what you do known to them.

Public relations

This is a way for therapists to get their name in the public eye without actually paying for advertising.

There is a variety of ways in which it can be done.

1 Offering a free talk and demonstration to a particular client group in the community is an ideal way of marketing Indian Head Massage and helping to get your name and reputation established Public interest in holistic therapies is increasing all the time and there are many groups that meet regularly who may be keen to hear from you (a list of contact names, addresses and phone numbers may be obtained from your local library).
See Talks and demonstrations (preceding page).

2 Sending information or news concerning your business to editors of newspapers or magazines in the form of a news article. Every day, editors and journalists are looking for stories and information to fill their newspapers or magazines.
An important consideration when sending information to journalists is to send only information that is truly of interest to the community and their readers.

3 Donating your time, money or products to a local worthwhile charity. There are many charitable organisations who rely on donations each year in order to survive. An event linked to funding or sponsoring a charity would be a newsworthy article, as well as helping to meet the needs of the community.

4 Getting a regular or one-off slot on local radio (*see* local radio, page 236).

5 Compiling a press release which may be sent to local and national newspapers and magazines. When compiling a press release the following guidelines may help to increase your chance of publication:
• think of an original, interesting, thought-provoking or even humorous headline
• avoid trying to sell your service
• it should be newsworthy and of interest to the journalists and their readers
• address the information directly to a named editor or journalist, preferably one with whom you have already established contact
• ensure that it is laid out clearly (preferably double-line spacing) and is no longer than two pages
• always include a contact name, address and telephone number.

> ### *key note*
>
> Editorials in newspapers and magazines are seen to be credible and true as readers place a considerable amount of trust in the objectivity of journalists. It is therefore worth getting to know editors and journalists and being persistent, as the articles they write tend to hold a lot of weight with readers.

Indirect approach to marketing and promotion

There are several other methods of advertising or marketing which may be used in order to reach the potential clients you cannot reach in person, and these include:

*   newspaper advertising
*   specialist magazines
*   national directories
*   mailshots
*   leaflets and promotional material
*   the Internet
*   local radio
*   cross merchandising promotional literature.

Advertising strategies usually involve a mix of different media and should be scheduled over a period of time for maximum effect. Isolated advertisements rarely sustain enough interest.

Advertising is about getting your message across. Important considerations when considering an advertisement are:

*   what do you want to say to potential clients?
*   who is your target audience?
*   how will you communicate to them what you want to say?

It is essential to follow the tried and tested **AIDA** formula when considering your publicity:

A – attracting **ATTENTION** – this can be created by an appropriate heading that attracts attention
I – generating **INTEREST** – this can be created by stating what is on offer
D – creating **DESIRE** – this can be created by stating why what you have to offer is needed and getting potential clients to believe in the benefits
A – motivating **ACTION** – this can be created by offering the reader an incentive (special offer).

Good advertisements are usually targeted to the right audience, accurate and not misleading, catchy, concise and memorable. Effective adverts must have a good headline (select a major benefit for this) to have immediate impact. A good headline will:

*   attract the reader's attention
*   compel the person to read further

231

- improve response
- express the most important benefits.

A good advert should be easy to read and be written to:

- touch people's emotions
- be informative
- promote the service
- raise awareness
- motivate the reader to act.

When designing adverts, ask yourself what adverts you responded to and why.

> *key note*
>
> Words that tend to sell in adverts include:
>
> You, New, Results, Health, Free, Complimentary, Benefits, Now, Yes.

Local papers

There are two types of advertisements in newspapers and these are display advertisements and business classified. Display advertising is more expensive and could appear anywhere in the paper, unless you have paid to have a particular space such as the front or back page, or the television page (any of which could prove very expensive).

It is always a gamble when relying on display advertising as it may be largely dependent on the following:

- the day of the week the paper is printed
- the time of the year
- the page the advert appears on
- the layout of the advert in relation to the other advertisers.

An important point to consider with display advertising is that people buy papers for many reasons other than to read adverts (reading news, announcements and events, crosswords, horoscope). It is therefore important to consider how your advert is going to grab their attention, bearing in mind that newspapers have a short life-span, and bearing in mind also the AIDA principle.

It is also useful to consider that the person reading the news and features may come across your display advert and may not be thinking about a massage until he or she sees your advert, or they may not be ready to have a massage for some while. In fact it may take many exposures to your advert before this person feels you are sufficiently familiar to give you a try. It is important therefore that adverts are repeated regularly in the same way in order to create familiarity. It can also help to have a picture of yourself in the advert as it will be more eye-catching and will help the potential client to feel they know you.

It is important to remember when writing adverts that you are speaking directly to your potential clients and the reader will be initially attracted by your headline message, rather than the name of your business. It is often helpful to give the reader a reason to reply now, such as a deadline on a special offer, as this motivates action.

When you have designed an advert, it is often helpful to ask friends and colleagues to cast an eye over the design and the wording for critical review; often, a fresh pair of eyes can help add constructive comments.

Display advertising is usually more effective when it is combined with some editorial. Often papers run special features on health-related matters and it may be more appropriate to consider a display advert within a feature as it draws the reader's attention to a more focused subject. Classified advertising is more cost-effective than display advertising as it is more targeted to the service to be provided. The disadvantage with classified is that there may not always be an appropriate section for holistic therapists and advertising will need to be placed frequently in order to make it effective.

Specialist magazines

These are usually targeted to a specific audience and the ones related to health are those normally of interest to a holistic therapist. The main drawback with them is that they are not local but national and will depend on the readership and the location of the therapist as to whether the advertising will be effective.

> ### key note
> Check the readership profile before committing to advertising in magazines and check circulation radius and readership numbers.

Promotional material

When writing and designing promotional material the key to success is to write it as if you know the client personally. Choose words carefully in order that they strike a chord with the client. Remember that many clients reading promotional material may not know they are looking for your service until they see it.

It is also important when developing marketing material to ensure that it reflects the image you wish to portray and that it appeals to the target market.

Promotional materials such as leaflets, brochures and posters are the means by which clients will decide whether to contact you for an appointment. Promotional material must be attractive enough to make clients read it and wording should be positive, direct and above all personal. Brochures and posters with a question and answer format can help clients to overcome their objections and visual aids can help to attract attention.

It is also important to use positive language and turn a negative statement (such as a client's problem) into a positive one (how your treatment is going to help them). Including testimonials from satisfied clients (with their permission) can also help to build credibility and break down barriers.

233

Mailshots

Mailshots can be a worthwhile exercise but require a degree of planning and forethought. It is far more effective to target a specific group when designing a mailshot, as the main theme is to address the needs of all the respondents.

You may choose to target self-help groups with a common need of relaxation or to write to the Occupational Health Adviser at local companies, offering to give free talks and demonstrations as part of their stress management programme.

The letter should be sent on headed notepaper and be brief and concise. The focus should be on the respondent's needs, although it is helpful to send background information on yourself along with information on Indian Head Massage.

Mailshots usually have a success or response rate of around 2 per cent, although this may be enhanced to 5 per cent by follow-up phone calls.

> ### *key note*
> When writing to companies it is worth offering the incentive of corporate membership, as a promotion to motivate more clients to use your service. Each employee may be issued with a corporate membership card which entitles them to a certain percentage discount.

When sending a mailshot it is important to consider the day it is mailed out as this could have a significant effect on the result. If sending a mailshot to clients' homes, aim to send it to arrive on a Friday or Saturday, ready for the weekend, when they may have more time to consider what you are offering. If sending mailshots to companies, aim to send the information to arrive on a Tuesday or Wednesday and not on a Friday or Monday.

Getting corporate clients

Indian Head Massage is ideally suited to the workplace because of its unique selling points:
* it is portable in nature
* it is quick
* it provides a solution to the client's problems
* it is a personal service
* there is no need for the client to undress
* no special resources are required.

If your objective is to secure contracts with corporate clients, first consider which companies (both large and small) are within your catchment area and the profile of the staff members.

When approaching corporate clients, it is important to create a corporate image for yourself, even if you are not part of a large organisation. The first point of contact should be by letter directly to the person within the organisation who is responsible for the health and welfare of staff (this may be an Occupational Health Adviser, Staff Nurse, Health and Safety Officer, or Managing Director). The letter should be sent on quality headed notepaper; the main theme of the letter should be focused on the workplace benefits of Indian Head Massage and how it can benefit the staff and the organisation (see stress management chapter). When approaching corporate clients it is advisable to avoid 'flowery' therapy language and be specific and accurate in terms of the outcome (the benefits). Offer to come in and give a free talk and demonstration with no obligation. Once the letter has been sent, keep a record of it and follow it up with a phone call approximately seven to ten days afterwards.

Remember that businesses, whether large or small, receive a lot of paperwork through the post. Do not assume that the reason you have not heard from them is that they are not interested. They may simply not have had the time to read your letter.

Publications and directories

Advertising in national publications and directories such as Yellow Pages can be an effective way of advertising, as it is targeted to a specific skill area by virtue of the fact it is classified by therapy type. It is also a long-term form of advertising and can prove to be cost-effective as many are yearly publications.

Therapists should also consider their geographical location; if they are situated between two counties, it may be advisable to take an advert in more than one directory.

If there are several therapists advertising under the same category then it is important to consider your USP (Unique Sellling Point) and stress this in order to give a point of difference from competitors.

Internet

Some therapists are now taking advantage of the Internet as a means of advertising their treatments. An attractively designed web page including a treatment menu and a photograph of the therapist can all be factors that may enhance contact from any interested parties. It can also help to give a therapist a more corporate image, which is especially important if it is this sector of the market you are interested in pursuing.

Some feel that the Internet is a little impersonal but others who are constantly using it feel it is a very effective means of communication.

It is certainly worth considering this as a potential source of enquiries and contact, but remember that not everyone will have access to the Internet and many may prefer the more traditional means of contact.

Radio

Radio is an excellent form of media in raising awareness of treatments such as Indian Head Massage. Consider contacting your local radio station with a view to having either a regular or one-off spot on the radio to promote Indian Head Massage. It is important when approching the station to make the proposal interesting and one which will interest their listeners. It is important to respond to local trends or issues (for instance lifestyle or reducing stress) when presenting information on the radio, as it has to be topical and of value to listeners. Assessing growth trends within the industry will help you to assess the opportunities afforded to you.

When preparing to talk on the radio it is important to find out as much as possible about the programme you will be appearing on, the profile of the listeners and most importantly the style of the radio presenter. Some presenters prefer to work to a script and will run through a list of questions before the programme; others prefer to work unscripted and make the presentation more spontaneous.

> ## key note
>
> Local radio stations often look for gifts that can be given to listeners in exchange for on-air promotions. Donating your services is an easy and effective way of getting your name out on the airwaves without buying advertising time.

Cross-merchandising promotional literature

Consider other local businesses that cater to clientele similar to yours (e.g. hairdressers, osteopaths etc.) and who may be in a position to influence clients to try Indian Head Massage.

Exchange promotional literature and brochures with them and this will allow each party additional exposure to the type of clients they wish to attract. When approaching other local businesses with a view to cross-merchandising, it is important to establish a friendly, approachable and co-operative working relationship, as this will enhance the success of the promotion on both sides.

Encouraging client retention

The first goal of marketing is to encourage potential clients to try out your services; the next goal is to encourage them to come back again. There are several ways of fostering repeat business:

- creating an understanding of the benefits of the treatments you provide to clients by encouraging them to book regular treatments
- awarding loyalty bonuses and reward schemes (such as ones offered by major supermarket chains)
- staying in touch with your clients and informing them of special offers and any new treatments you may have added to your treatment menu (and how these can benefit them)
- inviting clients to attend talks and events you may be holding.

Maximising marketing opportunities

Because of the widespread appeal of Indian Head Massage it is well suited to clinics, salons and spas, as well as other associated trades such as hairdressers, osteopaths, chiropractors and health clinics. Consider all places where people attend regularly for reasons of health, beauty and relaxation.

A local hairdresser's may be interested in adding Indian Head Massage to their treatment menu to give a different marketing angle to their customer service.

Osteopaths and chiropractors may be interested in Indian Head Massage for clients with soft-tissue problems of the head, neck and shoulders.

A GP surgery may be interested in helping clients with stress, anxiety and depression or people with musculo–skeletal problems.

If you have a local regional airport nearby, they may be interested in a business proposal to offer treatments to tired business executives in need of stress relief.

A local school may benefit from a regular visit to help teachers and students to manage their stress levels.

If you use your imagination, there is a multitude of different opportunities and reasons for marketing Indian Head Massage.

Selling of associated products

As providing treatments is a labour-intensive service, consider selling complementary products for clients' home use. Clients are more likely to buy products such as scalp oils and relaxation tapes at the time of their treatment. It is therefore advisable to have a display of items available for purchase at reception or wherever the client is likely to pay. Clients are also more likely to buy from their therapist, with whom they have a trusting relationship.

Creative marketing opportunities

Other creative marketing opportunities could be to offer gift certificates linked to promotions at specific times of the year such as Christmas, Valentine's Day, birthdays, Mother's Day or Father's Day. Specially packaged courses of treatment often attract interest as they are designed specifically to address the needs of the respondents.

Male clients

An area that is often left unexploited is the market of male clients. Marketing treatments such as Indian Head Massage can require a different strategy from selling to female clients.

Men often respond more to factual and benefit-related words rather than the more kinaesthetic language women tend to respond to. Think of male-dominated markets and how that target may be reached. Local sports clubs and associations may be a good start; also men's barbers, health clubs.

An important consideration when marketing to male clients is to consider whether the environment you are practising in is male-friendly (it will be difficult to attract male clients into a salon that looks too pretty). Some men are also conscious of their body image; it may therefore be more prudent to schedule specific times for male clients to attend.

Defining Marketing Objectives

Once you have put together the right mix of marketing methods, the next stage is to define your marketing objectives. Marketing objectives are closely linked to overall business objectives and will define what you want to achieve from your marketing and how you intend to meet the objectives.

Example of marketing objectives for a therapist practising Indian Head Massage:

Objectives

Short term
1   To introduce Indian Head Massage to existing clientele

Medium term
2   To expand the existing client base to secure new clients

Long term
3   To introduce Indian Head Massage into the workplace

Strategy

1   Send a newsletter to all existing clients advising them of the benefits of Indian Head Massage and how it can help them. Include a voucher with a special introductory offer.

2   Contact the editor of a local newspaper to offer an article on Indian Head Massage that is going to be of interest to readers, and a free demonstration.

3   Write to 20 local companies with a short but informative introductory letter. Offer a corporate discount. Follow up with a phone call in seven to ten days with a view to securing a meeting to offer a free talk and demonstration.

Monitoring marketing methods

It is important to regularly monitor the response to marketing methods, to help you assess which methods are working to help you meet your business objectives.

It is essential to constantly monitor, review and adapt your strategies in order to ensure continued business success. Marketing methods may change with a difference in trend or may simply become out-dated.

A simple and effective way of monitoring the response to your marketing methods is to ask each new client how they heard of you and keep a record of this in order to review it in line with your business objectives. Provided you know how much a particular method cost and how many clients were generated from it, you are then in a position to analyse which methods are cost-effective.

Once you establish a clientele you can then build up information such as how often they attend for treatments, how much they spend and what marketing methods they respond to.

For marketing to have the desired effects it should be:

*   **SUFFICIENT** – it has to be done regularly, even when you are busy
*   **EFFICIENT** – it has to be cost-effective to be worthwhile
*   **EFFECTIVE** – it has to work and get results.

How to Encourage Repeat Business

Maintaining excellent customer service is the key to encouraging repeat business.

It is important to make it easy for clients to come to you by:

- making client needs a priority
- concentrating all your actions and efforts for the business with the client in mind
- treating every client like a new client and avoiding complacency
- delivering an excellent service
- building an open relationship with clients by encouraging feedback.

Keeping ahead of business

Many businesses fail to realise their potential because they don't continually market themselves. An important factor to consider is that many clients may have to see your advert or marketing material many times before responding.

Many therapists fail to be consistent in marketing methods, believing they already have enough clients. Even if the appointment book is full, it is important to keep on marketing to raise client awareness and maintain your professional image, as you never know when you are going to lose current clients because of various circumstances (client's personal or financial circumstances, client moving out of the area etc.).

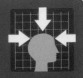

activity task

Design a Marketing Plan for Indian Head Massage based on the following outline:

1 Description of the service to be offered (i.e. Indian Head Massage)

Include your unique selling points (USPs) and a full description of the service and how it can benefit clients

2 Objectives of the marketing campaign

This could be to increase your client market, or to raise awareness of Indian Head Massage etc.

3 A profile of your intended client market

This is whom you want to target and why you think they will pay for the service. Include as much information as possible, based on what you have discovered about your potential clients (market questionnaires, interviews etc.). Also include information on competitors, if applicable, as this will help you to identify how much your potential clients are currently spending on a similar service.

4 Where you intend to offer the service (location)

Because of its portability, consider the different locations in which Indian Head Massage treatment may be offered

5 Details of your SWOT analysis

(strengths, weaknesses, opportunities, threats)

6 Intended marketing strategies

Consider how you intend to advertise the service, what media you will use and how often you will advertise
Consider all the direct and indirect forms of marketing and promotions that will help your business succeed
Design a promotional leaflet for Indian Head Massage
Remember to allocate a budget for marketing activities and to plan the activities out over a period of time for maximum effect

BIBLIOGRAPHY AND FURTHER READING

Ashley, Martin
Massage – A career at your fingertips
Enterprise Publishing (1999)
ISBN 0 9644662 6 0

Bennett, Ruth
The Science of Beauty Therapy
Hodder & Stoughton (1995)
ISBN 0 340 63079 5

Burton, J.L.
Essentials of Dermatology
Churchill Livingstone (1985)
ISBN 0 443 03100 2

Caldwell, Diane
Marketing Campaigns
International Thomson Publishing (1998)
ISBN 1 86152 245 2

Cox, Gill and Dainow, Sheila
Making the Most of Yourself
Sheldon Press (1988)
ISBN 0 85969 178 X

Falloon, Val
How to Get More Clients
BPCC Wheatons Ltd, Exeter (1992)
ISBN 0 9513347 5 1

Fry, Lionel
Dermatology – An Illustrated Guide (Second edition)
Update Publications Ltd
ISBN 0 906141 02 8

Gardner-Gordon, Joy
Pocket Guide to Chakras
Vibrational Healing Enterprises (1998)
ISBN 0 89594 949 0

Gaudin, Anthony J. and Jones, Kenneth C.
Human Anatomy & Physiology
Harcourt Brace (1989)
ISBN 0 15 539705 2

Harland, Madeleine and Finn, Glen
Healthy Business – The Natural Practitioner's Guide to Success
Hyden House Ltd (1990)
ISBN 1 85623 000 7

Hole Jr, J. W.
Human Anatomy and Physiology
William C. Brown Publishers (1993)
ISBN 0 697 12271 9

Gill, Jit
Stress Survival Guide
HarperCollins Publishers (Collins Gem) (1999)
ISBN 0 00 472321 X

Harish, Johari
Ancient Indian Massage – Traditional Massage Techniques Based on the Ayurveda
Munshiram Manoharlal Publishers Pvt. Ltd. (1997 edition – originally published 1984)
ISBN 81 215 0008 7

MacKie, Rona M.
Clinical Dermatology
Oxford University Press (1991, reprinted 1993)
ISBN 0 19 261980 2

McGuinness, Helen
Anatomy & Physiology – Beauty Therapy Basics
Second Edition
Hodder & Stoughton Educational (2002)
ISBN 0 340 80208 1

Mehta, Narendra
Indian Head Massage
Thorsons (1999)
ISBN 0 7225 3791 3

Mernagh-Ward, Dawn and Cartwright, Jennifer
Good Practice in Salon Management
Stanley Thornes (1997)
ISBN 0 7487 2887 2

Oxford Concise Colour Medical Dictionary
Market House Books Ltd
Oxford University Press (1998)
ISBN 0 19 270085 X

Phillips, Carol
In the Bag – Selling in the Salon
Milady Salon Ovations (1995)
ISBN 1 56253 236 7

Premkumar, Kalyani
Pathology A to Z
VanPub Books (1996)
ISBN 0 9680730 0 X

Record, Matthew
Preparing a Business Plan
How to Books Ltd, Oxford (1998)
ISBN 1 85703 374 4

Sachs, Melanie
Ayurvedic Beauty Care
Lotus Press (1994)
ISBN 0 914955 11 X

Salvo, Susan G.
Massage Therapy – Principles & Practice
W.B. Saunders Company (1999)
ISBN 0 7216 7419 4

Sharamon, Shalila and Baginski, Bodo J.
The Chakra Handbook
Lotus Light Publications (1997)
ISBN 0 941524 85 X

Tortora and Grabowski
Principles of Anatomy and Physiology
Harper Collins (1992)
ISBN 0 06 046702 9

White, Dr Adrian
Stress and Anxiety (Help Yourself to Health)
Godsfield Press Ltd
ISBN 1 899434 38 0

Wilkinson, J.D. and Shaw, S.
Dermatology (A Colour Guide)
Churchill Livingstone (1987)
ISBN 0 443 05852 0

Williams, Sara
Lloyds Bank Small Business Guide
Penguin Books (1997)
ISBN 0 14 026836 7

Resource Section

For professional training courses, training videos and posters, contact:

The Holistic Training Centre
Abacus House
1 Spring Crescent
Portswood
Southampton
SO17 2FZ
(02380) 390982
e-mail: info@holistictrainingcentre.co.uk

For a selection of authentic Indian massage and hair oils, contact:

Maharishi Ayur-Veda Products
Beacon House
Willow Walk
Skelmersdale
Lancs
WN8 6UR
(01695) 51015
e-mail: dwhitley@maharishi.co.uk

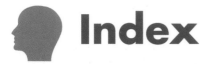

Index